...ɴɢ CHRONIC PAIN THROUGH YOGA

The Therapeutic Art of Mindful Movement

QAT WANDERS

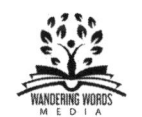

WANDERING WORDS
MEDIA

Copyright © 2018 Qat Wanders, Wandering Words Media. All rights reserved.

No part of this publication may be reproduced, distributed, or transmitted in any form or by any means, including photocopying, recording, or other electronic or mechanical methods, without the prior written permission of the publisher, except in the case of brief quotations embodied in reviews and certain other noncommercial uses permitted by copyright law.

Published by Wandering Words Media 2018 www.WanderingWordsMedia.com

Cover design by www.100covers.com

Editor: Shanique Carter

Proofreader: Mario Jacobs

Formatter: Ramanathan Perumal

PRAISE FOR QAT WANDERS

"*Overcoming Chronic Pain Through Yoga* takes a unique approach to education. On the one hand, it reads like you are learning from an authority on health and wellness and at the same time, it also feels like you are having a conversation with a close friend who is trying to help you get healthier while hanging out on your couch on a Sunday afternoon.

Qat gives you the details if you want them, but also simply tells you what you can do. I love her personal stories of struggle and victory that she eloquently explains throughout the book. This is a must-read for anyone looking to improve their health!"

~Dr. Jason Piken DC, CNS, author of *Better!: 11 Simple Habits to Improve Your Life*

"Highly Recommended Book In Overcoming Chronic Pain

"This book is a treasure to keep. One should have this book as it offers excellent, practical and doable tips for overcoming chronic pain. This is not just about the yoga that everyone knows: spandex and headstands. It is much better than this. What makes this book a more interesting read is how the author shared her own chronic pain experiences, how she dealt with it, what she learned and discovered, what worked and did not work in eradicating her pain, and then generously and lovingly provided tips that can EFFECTIVELY help people. I love the tips on Mindfulness and Shifting Mindset just to name a few. These should be the foundation of all healing modalities. Be healed and get this book now!"

~Elsa Mendoza, Best-Selling Author of *YOU CAN QUOTE ME ON THIS: Words to Empower You and Awaken Your Consciousness*

"Finally! An easily digestible how-to manual for anyone who is looking to overcome their chronic pain and regain control of their life, health, and overall well-being. Qat Wanders has a compelling backstory worthy of writing this book of deep knowledge for people needing to overcome their suffering and as she points out, overcome fear. If you are in constant anticipation of experiencing your chronic pain and live in fear of it, don't waste another second and buy this book. Because if you are willing to have dedication, motivation, faith, and a strong belief that you actually can get better, then this book will be your new must-read."

~ **Sarah Saint-Laurent, Certified Wellness Coach and Best-Selling Author of** *Awakening Sexy Shakti*

"Qat Wanders' book *Overcoming Chronic Pain Through Yoga,* gets my highest recommendation for anyone dealing with chronic pain.

"I work as the lead Physical Therapist for one of the nation's top Spine Centers in Sacramento, California where I am working with pain management doctors, surgeons, therapists, acupuncturists and other medical staff to help those that are dealing with chronic pain. And I am always looking for the best resources for my patients; this will now be at the top of my list.

"The content is easy to read and shows how all the different systems in your body can contribute to your pain, including concepts like hypermobility, fibromyalgia, sciatica and repetitive trauma. She also has specific actions that you can take to not only understand your body's symptoms, but to start treating them, including her own Mindful Movement Techniques. As she talks about in the book, Qat does not only have the education and experience of working with people in chronic pain, but has experienced it herself and knows what it takes to get back to a life where you are not limited by pain.

"I will be using this as a tool to help my patients dealing with pain of all types including long-lasting chronic pain, and would highly recommend it for anyone who is currently living their lives in the shadow of chronic pain."

~Sean Sumner
Physical Therapist, Orthopedic Clinical Specialist, Lead PT at The Spine Center at UC Davis Medical Center, Author of the best-selling book, *Sciatica, and the Super Spine Series*

CONTENTS

Introduction	xv
1. How to Use This Book	1
2. What is Your WHY?	7
3. Why I Do What I Do	13
4. Adopting Mindfulness	37
5. Shifting Mindset	49
6. Are You Dependent on Painkillers?	61
7. Emotional Chronic Pain	67
8. Getting to Know YOU	79
9. Ayurveda in a Nutshell	83
10. Acid vs Alkaline	91
11. Yoga with Subcategories	127
12. Hot Yoga	143
13. The Body Is A Temple So What Went WRONG!?	145
14. Metabolic Reconditioning	169
15. Technique #1	179
16. Technique #2	185
17. Technique #3	189
18. Technique #4	193
19. Now Let's Keep the Brain Healthy	197
20. Chronic Pain While Traveling	201
21. End-of-Life Pain	207
22. Allowing the Transformation to Happen	213
Afterword	219
23. Gut-Healing Diet Sample Recommendation	221
About the Author	227
Also by Qat Wanders	230
Acknowledgments	233
24. Resources	235

To my daughter, Ora, who gave me the reason and motivation to overcome chronic pain in the first place!

The stories and suggestions offered in this book are based entirely upon the author's personal experience, and the experiences of the author's clients.

The information provided in this book is designed to provide helpful information on the subjects discussed. This book is not meant to be used to diagnose or treat any medical condition. The author is not responsible for any specific health needs that may require medical supervision and is not liable for any damages or negative consequences from any action, to any person reading or following the information in this book. References are provided for informational purposes only and do not constitute endorsement of any websites or other sources. Readers should be aware that the websites listed in this book may change.

Yoga - More than Exercise

"Yoga says the body is the vehicle for the soul, but no one ever washes a rented car."

— ~B.K.S. IYENGAR

INTRODUCTION

"It is not *normal* to be sick. It is *common* to be sick. But our bodies can heal until we interfere."

— KIMBERLY MASKA

Millions of people today are suffering silently (or not so silently) from chronic pain. This pain can come in so many forms and on so many different levels of severity. For some, it's an *invisible illness*. These people don't even look sick, but they are suffering on a daily basis. For others, their pain is obvious, and they are dealing with not only physical pain but the emotional affiliations of having people feel sorry for them, stare at them, and talk to them with pity in their eyes.

Chronic pain affects lives negatively on many levels.

INTRODUCTION

The repercussions are more than just physical. It leads to tremendous mental and spiritual problems as well. When we suffer, especially if we feel we are suffering pointlessly and endlessly, it creates a vicious loop of emotions that make us feel hopeless, angry, and miserable.

But what if someone were to tell you there is a way to overcome this suffering on a physical, emotional, and spiritual level? A method that doesn't involve spending hundreds or thousands of dollars every month on expensive medications or supplements for the rest of your life?

In this book, I'm going to show you the exact method I used to overcome the chronic pain that took over my life for almost 30 years. These techniques have helped not only me overcome chronic pain, but hundreds of my students as well.

As a licensed Yoga Therapist, Ayurvedic Specialist, and Integrative Medicine Practitioner, I have dedicated the last 10 years of my life to helping others overcome chronic pain because I know what type of suffering they are going through. I know how much this can affect everyday life. And it has been a slow process, but I developed the Mindful Movement Techniques™ which help trigger the body's pain responses in a way that can help overcome chronic pain quickly and effectively. On top of these physical movements, there are multiple life-style adjustments as well which have proven effective for literally everyone I have worked with.

INTRODUCTION

Because of these techniques, my students are having great success. They have been able to take back control of their lives and their health and move through the world with more energy and optimism.

The best part about these techniques is that you can implement them immediately. Tyson, a client from Kansas, says, "I can't believe how quickly I noticed results! I am not even having spasms since we started working together for crying out loud..."

I promise you that if you follow the steps and fully implement what you learn in this book, and make it a true part of your lifestyle, you are going to have more energy, better mental clarity, less pain, and less stress.

You will have the ability to involve yourself more with your family, your friends, your relationships, and your life. Work will become easier, your attitude and outlook on life will become more pleasant, and you will be able to look back down the path of healing that you have been slowly walking on and realize you have made it further than you ever thought possible.

Don't be the type of person who uses your pain and suffering as an excuse for getting sympathy from others. Be the type of person who takes control of your own life and health. Be the type of person who others look to for motivation and inspiration, who can look back and say "I was serious and motivated about transforming my body and health, and I'm so glad I did it—because look at me now!"

What a beautiful way to help others.

INTRODUCTION

The tips and techniques you will read about in this book have been proven to create positive, effective, and long-lasting results. All you have to do is approach these methods with an open mind and motivation, and you will be amazed by your progress. Get ready to look in the mirror and see a whole new version of you. When we can live our lives free from the control that chronic pain has over us, we can truly live as the best versions of ourselves.

So what are you waiting for? Jump in right now. Allow yourself the gift of new experiences and perspectives. You deserve it.

HOW TO USE THIS BOOK

I want to be very clear here when I tell you that as I talk about Yoga, I am not, in any way, talking about putting on tight pants and turning yourself into a pretzel. Although I do focus heavily on the physical Yoga postures in this book—for the purpose of learning how to overcome chronic pain—the title of this book, *Overcoming Chronic Pain Through Yoga,* refers to the spiritual science of Yoga itself.

So, if you were expecting a technical book full of pictures of people in spandex showing you how to stand on your head, then you are in the *wrong* place.

You are in the *right* place, however, if you are interested in improving your physical, mental, and spiritual fitness level. Or, if you have an open mind, and you are serious and motivated about achieving transformational healing.

This book is not for the faint of heart. It is intended

for those who are done suffering and ready to move forward with their lives on all levels and be the best possible versions of themselves they can be.

So if that is you, keep reading. I have set this book up in a particular sequence for a reason. You may just be itching to get to the Mindful Movement Techniques™, but they are placed toward the end of the book for a very specific purpose. So please read through this book *in order.*

I recommend either reading all the way through and then going back through it again to implement things one by one or take your time going through this book one section at a time. Once you are comfortable with each thing, and you have tried it out, then move forward.

Let me repeat: *this book is sequential!*

I would also like to point out, that if you happen to be in such a situation that any sort of physical activity is absolutely unobtainable for you, you can still do all the physical practices **in your mind.** It may sound a bit ridiculous, but give it a shot, because if something is not *physically* possible, it is still *mentally* possible. And in time this will lead to it being physically possible for you as well.

Initially, I intended for this to be the manual to supplement my Pain-Free Life Program. But as I got further in depth, I decided to make two different variations. That is how this particular book that you are holding came to be. It is still a companion to my Pain-

Free Life Program, but it has been simplified to be read all the way through by anyone—even if they aren't working with me directly.

Each chapter in this book is designed to give you new insights you can apply directly to multiple areas of your life. I have personally used them in my own life and have seen positive and long-lasting results.

I recommend bookmarking or highlighting the sections of this book that you feel would be helpful for your own personal situation. That way, you can come back to them after you have read the whole book. You can also try these techniques as you go along. If you think it is something you should try, go ahead and try it out and pay attention to the results. Most importantly, pay attention to how it makes you *feel*.

If your body is resisting something, there is a reason for that. But frequently, our minds resist something and try to convince us it is really our bodies that are resisting. So pay attention. Is it your *mind* resisting, or your *body?*

If your mind is resisting, try to assess why. If you can fully understand what it is your mind has an aversion to, it can help you overcome and learn to accept the physical and emotional sensations that are brought up.

I will give you as much helpful information as I possibly can in this book. I want to offer everyone this information, and although I wish I could work one-on-one with every single one of you, I am limited by the fact that there is only one of me. But I have worked hard to put together a framework you can follow yourself and use to structure your own personal practice.

So what is it I did exactly? What are these techniques? Well, it took me a really long time to figure it out. But I am excited to share them with you!

Overcome: *verb* over·come \ ˌō-vər-ˈkəm \ overcoming;

    1:to get the better of :SURMOUNT

    overcome difficulties

    : to successfully deal with or gain control of (something difficult)

— MERRIAM-WEBSTER.COM

WHAT IS YOUR WHY?

Why did I write this book? I wrote it because I spent almost 30 years dealing with debilitating chronic pain. It affected my life negatively in more ways than I could even count. It left me feeling utterly hopeless, useless, and burdensome to everyone around me.

I was dependent entirely upon painkillers to function as a human being, and it made me hate myself. This led to mental issues as well, such as suicidal depression and resentment toward God and the others around me who weren't dealing with the kind of pain I was.

Once I started getting better, people kept asking me how I did it. Everyone wanted to know what my fantastic secret was. What was the magic bullet that helped me overcome chronic pain?

I realized that I was onto something, and I wanted to help others as well. Now that I can say I have completely overcome chronic pain—meaning it doesn't affect my life negatively anymore—I have made it my personal mission to help as many people as possible who have suffered similarly.

But the truth is; *there is no magic bullet*. It's a process. And the process looks different for everyone. It is possible—it just takes dedication, motivation, and faith in yourself. As well as a strong belief that you actually *can* get better!

This is my *why*. This is why I wrote this book. This is why I created my program. To help others help themselves.

I know my process works because I have seen it change lives. So, needless to say, I am more than a little bit excited to share this information with you here. I realize, of course, there is only so much I can do in the form of a book. But I did my best to compile everything I teach my clients right here into these pages. That's it.

This is my everything. I'm not trying to sell you some course or program at the end. I'm letting it all hang out here. So, I would like to offer it up to the world as my humble attempt to make this world a better place—a place with a little less suffering.

Now let's talk about YOU. Why are you here? Why did you pick up this book? Pardon me for making an assumption, but I'm going to go ahead and venture to guess that you are reading this because you have been dealing with chronic pain for at least a somewhat extended period. This chronic pain has probably affected your life in more ways than you even realize. Or maybe you *do* realize it, and that makes you want to make these changes even more!

I am also going to assume that because you saw the word *overcoming* in the title, you are ready—in some sense—to overcome chronic pain and move forward on a healing path that will help you regain control of your life and health.

Now, I'm going to ask you to look a little bit deeper. What is your *why?* Why do you want to overcome chronic pain? There are a lot of levels to this question.

On the surface level it probably seems obvious. You want to stop suffering. But let's go a little deeper than that. Why exactly do you want to stop suffering? Is it because the pain is making you feel hopeless and useless? Do you feel like a burden on your friends and family?

Is it because you're so dependent on painkillers to keep the pain at bay that it's turning you into a zombie? Do you feel incoherent and miserable?

Is the pain making you so irritable or angry that you are snapping at your loved ones and then feeling guilty about it later on?

Could it be that you had to stop doing the things you love, and now your life feels meaningless and empty?

Maybe it's because you can't even get out of bed in the morning without reaching for the bottle of Vicodin (or perhaps it's just ibuprofen, which is actually just as detrimental—if not more so—to your stomach and digestive tract).

Are you dealing with severe Irritable Bowel Syndrome that is keeping you from being able to go out to dinner with your friends? Or such painful arthritis you can't even leave the house when it's cold outside?

Now let's turn things around here—think about how different your life would be if you could actually overcome all of this! What would change?

Perhaps you could finally make it to your children's baseball games that they've wanted you to come to for years. Maybe you and your spouse will be able to start having sex again at last. Perhaps you can actually make plans in advance to go out with your friends and not feel incredibly guilty for having to cancel them at the last minute because you are too sick to go out.

Now let's go even deeper. What would doing all these things really be able to change in your life? So now you can do more things. You can spend more time with the ones you care about. You can partake in activities you love. You can think straight and carry on a conversation. Are you happier?

Do you feel a greater sense of self-worth? Will this give you a sense of being a better friend, lover, or parent? Maybe a better employee/employer?

Since chronic pain can greatly affect our finances—causing us to miss so much work—would overcoming this allow you the ability to bring in a higher income, in turn, allowing you more freedom? Perhaps even giving you more confidence and security?

Just sit with this for a moment. When we overcome pain—the end-goal is to truly overcome suffering. To overcome fear. After all, ***fear is just the anticipation of future pain.*** Now just imagine what life would be like for you if you could truly transcend all these things. Once and for all. How different would your overall *being* be? What about your personality?

This type of comfortability and serenity will shift the way we can give and receive love.

If that isn't enough motivation for us to overcome chronic pain on all levels then I don't know what is.

Now read over these questions again. Which one resonates with you the most? What really gets you in the heart? Gives you goosebumps? Makes your fingertips tingle?

This is your why.

This is why you are ready and motivated and serious about overcoming chronic pain.

So every time you start to feel like you're struggling, if you feel like you can't do this, or if you want to give up because it's not working right away, I want you to go back to your why. Maybe even take it a step further, write it down and put it where you can see it every day. Remember why you are choosing to overcome something that has held you back in life—held you back from being the best version of you.

WHY I DO WHAT I DO

"One person's healing affects everyone on the planet, and it resonates all the way out into the universe."

— BRIGETTE PATTON, SOUL MASSAGES

I'm going to launch into my own personal story here. Now, if you have read my previous book, *Yoga for YOU,* then you already know a little bit about my personal story. If you aren't interested in hearing more or even if you haven't read the book, but have no interest in reading about my chronic pain experience throughout my own life, then I am telling you right now to skip ahead to the next chapter.

Consider yourself warned.

I have chosen to share my experience with you here because I have found it to be the most efficient way to relate with others on a human level. Your story is different from mine, but there may be some similarities as well. I hope that my struggles and accomplishments will give you something to relate to—as well as inspiration.

I had many physical issues from a young age. But people would look at me and tell me I looked perfectly healthy, so there couldn't be anything wrong with me! They couldn't understand the physical pain I was going through.

The problem with an "invisible illness" is that when you look healthy; other people have trouble understanding the possible magnitude of what you are experiencing. People have an easy time ignoring what they can't physically see.

I guarantee that if you had an *actual* knife sticking out of your rib cage (rather than just the physical sensation of the knife)—complete with blood oozing everywhere—then people would probably take your suffering pretty darn seriously and treat you with significantly more empathy!

People also told me that if I was actually doing Yoga then I would be healthier. Some didn't even believe I could be as dedicated to Yoga as I was. But the truth is, if I hadn't found Yoga, I would have been so much worse off. I don't even want to imagine where I would be now.

I spent so much of my life in chronic pain. I got my first migraine when I was two years old, and I had them about five times a week from then on. There were many days I couldn't even function. All I could do was lie in bed and wish I was dead. Not a great way to spend childhood.

I went through multiple migraine prescriptions. Various doctors. Nothing worked. I was finally told by a physician to just take over-the-counter pain relievers every single morning as soon as I woke up. I did that for over 20 years. But the migraines continued.

When I was 14, the debilitating sciatica started. Once again, I went to multiple doctors, and they discovered a torn nerve, but no one could figure out what had caused it. They told me that when I turned 18, they would be able to operate on me, but until then, all they could do was prescribe painkillers.

So at that point, the prescription painkillers also became part of my daily regimen. I had three different prescriptions because I had to switch them up regularly. If I took one kind for too long it stopped working, and the pain would get so excruciating I couldn't leave the house.

One doctor finally referred me to a physical therapist, but those sessions actually made the pain significantly worse, and I eventually stopped going after about six months. After that, I tried going to a chiropractor who was optimistic she would be able to help me—so I became hopeful as well.

But once again, the regular visits to the chiropractor (and I went three times per week, so I'm sure they absolutely loved the boatloads of money I was spending) also made my pain even worse.

The chiropractor, however, after looking at my x-rays, noticed a significant amount of arthritis in my spine and hips as well as my right wrist. I spent a lot of time writing and drawing, so my wrist was frequently sore, but I thought that was normal. They were so shocked by the amount of arthritis in such a young girl they sent me back to my primary care physician who then referred me to a rheumatologist.

The rheumatologist did little to help me—she really just informed me that the arthritis would be creeping through my body throughout my life and taking over my entire skeleton as time went on. And the pain would only get worse.

That isn't exactly what a high schooler wants to hear.

Just think, at this point, I was still a kid trying to enjoy my teenage years! You know those 'bomb-proof wonder years' that American teenagers just feel like they're so entitled to?

Yeah... I never got that.

As the pain progressed, I started looking into alternative methods to heal my body. I knew that I was too young to accept "It will only get worse," as a diagnosis.

Since books were my favorite thing in the world, I took to the libraries, used book stores, flea markets, and swap meets. That was how I discovered Yoga when I was 15. No one else was doing it. I had no guidance. My only instruction came from books.

The painkillers kept the problems at bay enough that I could function at an almost reasonable level. As long as I made sure to take them every four hours without fail, I was relatively all right.

If you know anything about painkillers—and what they do to the body—I'm sure you can only imagine what this has done to my stomach over the years.

I was about 18 when my digestive problems started getting pretty severe. I would suffer from gut-wrenching pain every time I ate. I went to every naturopath I could find because, at this point, I had lost all faith in Western medicine.

I have now had several doctors suggest surgery. I was also referred to two surgeons for operations on my lower back, surgery on my right wrist (because I supposedly had carpal tunnel), and now they were discussing the possibility of removing several feet of my intestines.

Hell no.

I had stated to all these doctors vehemently that I would not allow anyone to cut me open. I was adamant that I would be able to fix this myself. I just had to keep trying. First things first, I knew I desperately needed to get off the painkillers, but they were the only thing keeping me functional.

I was getting angrier and angrier at the world, and the suicidal thoughts were constant. I found it unfair that everyone else I knew got to live like normal human beings. They could walk around outside and talk to people and bend down without pain. I was beginning to doubt that I would ever know what that would be like. It was a feeling of utmost hopelessness.

As I got older, I started to study more of the science behind Yoga. I began to change my diet, my body products, and my environment. Meditation and spiritual practice didn't come until later, though.

I was practicing the physical Yoga postures daily and attending classes at several studios. I wanted to get to know all the different styles and figure out which worked best for me. They were all so different!

I apparently went a little bit overboard, though, because I had a major flare-up of brachial neuritis, which is a rare condition that affects several members of my family. It isn't necessarily painful, but it is certainly very inconvenient. It involves numbness and tingling and sometimes a small amount of pain coming from the brachial area in my shoulders.

By lifting my arms and tightening them over my head so often, I had aggravated it and lost complete feeling from my neck all the way down to my fingertips for several months. This was more aggravating than I could even tell you! I couldn't pick things up if they were heavier than about a half a pound, and I couldn't lift my arms above shoulder level at all. If I tried, that was when I felt pain.

But, because I was a teenager, I felt the need to keep pushing it. I kept telling myself if I just kept pushing my body I would eventually get better. *All it takes is willpower! Right?*

Not so much.

At 19, I decided to take matters completely into my own hands. I was practicing Yoga every single day, eating a ridiculously clean vegan diet, dancing professionally, and running competitively (thanks to the painkillers). And I thought this just made me so awesome.

On a whim, I decided to cut painkillers completely out of my life because they were so bad for me. So I went 'cold turkey.' However, this caused horrible repercussions. Not only did the pain come back in such monumental waves I can't even describe to you, but my body went into other drastic forms of withdrawal.

It was as if my brain just didn't work properly. I would get dizzy all the time. I had trouble understanding what people would say to me. I couldn't focus. I regularly saw floaters when I tried to look at any light source. On top of all that, I had horrible anxiety.

I read every book on natural healing I could get my hands on. I tried everything I could to reduce the migraines, arthritis, and sciatica—but nothing made even a slight dent in the pain.

At this point, I decided to enroll in an herbalism course in Northern California. I had to start taking the painkillers again just to do this, but I learned a tremendous amount from these brilliant teachers. This is where I was introduced to the concepts behind Ayurveda. I didn't even know what Ayurveda *was* before that. I thought I had just signed up for a course in herbal medicine.

Slowly, the concepts began to integrate into my way of life. I studied avidly. I knew that if I just kept studying, eventually, I would learn enough—and all the right things—to finally heal myself.

I wasn't dealing with just pain anymore, and I could tell there was a lot very wrong with my body. I could feel inside myself that my body wasn't working properly. I was downright toxic despite all of the actions I had taken to neutralize the toxic effects in my system.

I had terrible brain fog, mood swings, dizziness, and I occasionally lost consciousness without warning. I was rushed to the emergency room almost every month; sometimes by loved ones or even by strangers who saw me collapse.

Doctors had given me an assortment of diagnoses, but none of them could agree. On top of that, I frequently traveled, so I never had the same doctor.

But the one thing the doctors all agreed on, was that I had the skeleton of an 80-year-old. Doctors had been telling me that since I was 19. Frequently, when they looked at my x-rays, they thought it was a mistake—that they had gotten switched with someone's much older. *So embarrassing!*

As I got older things finally started to change. I studied Yoga, anatomy, and herbalism in more depth. I realized I had a talent for showing people how to do the postures and helping them find an awareness of their bodies. So I started teaching what I had learned to people I knew. And in 2008, I became a mother and also decided to become a certified Yoga teacher.

I had my certification in herbal medicine, and I was actively learning everything I could about human anatomy. I was collecting certifications like vintage stamps, but it wasn't until I got pregnant with my daughter that I began to figure some things out.

True to form, I spent my whole pregnancy doing prenatal Yoga postures and reading books about pregnancy. I wanted to fully understand the female body and exactly what it had to go through. I wanted to know every possible challenge I could face and anything I could do to prevent problems and make my situation easier.

All the health issues I had dealt with since adolescence became worse during my pregnancy. The migraines were worse than ever. The sciatica was continuously active. My spine and joints ached constantly. My digestion was almost at a complete standstill, and the brain fog and dizziness were so bad I could hardly do anything on my own. The pregnancy caused so much stress on my body that my mind became extremely stressed as well.

But once it was all said and done, I gave birth to a beautiful, perfectly healthy, baby girl who weighed almost 10 pounds. As I am sure you can imagine, this made everything worth it (though I doubt I will be doing it again—ever)!

After pregnancy, even though my health was worse than ever, my body bounced back impressively. I didn't have a single stretch mark, and I was back to my pre-pregnancy weight within two weeks.

I knew it was because of the Yoga.

People told me all the time how good I looked. However, I didn't *feel* good. Plus, after giving birth, I started having regular stomach pains.

I was no rookie to digestive issues. I had pretty severe stomach pains and cramps throughout the pregnancy. But every time I got examined, no one found anything wrong. So I finally learned to ignore it and just hoped it would get better afterward.

But it didn't get better. It got worse. A *lot* worse. Every time I ate, I experienced horrible, gripping pain (imagine gas pain times 50)! Every time I ate solid food, I became bloated and uncomfortable. My stomach would swell up, and I could hear my entire digestive tract gurgling as my food made its way through. I thought it was IBS (Irritable Bowel Syndrome), so I started looking into natural treatments for that.

It started to get a little bit better for a while, and then I tried cutting gluten out of my diet—which took the pain away completely. But this was only temporary (though I didn't know that at the time). I was so relieved to be rid of that horrible abdominal pain, I stayed on a gluten-free diet for years thinking I had solved the problem.

I kept up with my Yoga practice religiously. Any moment my daughter slept I used to practice the Yoga postures I had time for.

I did my best to stay in good physical shape. I rode my bike every day and even bought a jogging stroller and started running again.

I decided it was time for me to become a certified Yoga instructor. It seemed to me it was the only thing I would be able to do for a living. When I was practicing Yoga, I felt like a person. It was the only time I didn't feel completely sick. I could feel my body, and nourish my body, and treat it like the temple it truly was. But the rest of the day I felt ill. And even taking care of my baby was a huge challenge.

I made it through the teacher-training program in 2008 and received my official certification by the beginning of 2009. I had already been teaching for a couple of years at that point, but I wanted to have a real certification.

I started getting teaching jobs immediately. The program I went through my training with hired me upon my graduation and also helped me find other work. I quickly figured out that my niche was helping people who were dealing with chronic pain—specifically sciatica. I was able to use everything I had studied (and experienced) and put it to good use.

I continued to take more courses, get more certifications, and teach more classes of all different levels. But what I was best at was helping people with back problems. And those people didn't care how many certifications I had (I had Yoga Therapy, Integrative Medicine, and Ayurvedic Medicine certifications at this point as well). All they cared about was whether I could help them.

I had someone come to my Yoga class one day who came to talk to me afterward to tell me that his time in my class was the first time his chronic sciatica hadn't bothered him in months. We talked for quite a while about my own struggles with sciatica pain, and he was shocked; I didn't look like I was in any pain at all.

We decided to start doing one-on-one personal classes, and I was able to help him not just alleviate some of his pain, but eventually completely recover from the chronic sciatica he suffered from. The day I had met him he was walking with a cane, and after six months of working with me, he was competing in marathons again.

Not too shabby if you ask me!

I shifted my focus to helping students one on one. I began to realize that everyone's body was completely different. I knew that on a superficial level already, but working so closely with individuals made this clear.

I continued my study in anatomy, putting my herbalism knowledge somewhat on the back burner. I took on dozens of students who came to me with severe problems, and they were either completely cured or had their problems under control within six months. I was thrilled with how many people I was helping. I felt like I was doing something for the world, finally. But no matter how many people I was able to help, I still hadn't fixed myself.

After a while, I ended up getting burned out. I was teaching between 18 and 20 classes every week. Some of them were group classes, but most of them were individual. I was putting all my energy into helping others, while my own health progressively got worse. I was entirely reliant on painkillers to get me through the day. Every. Single. Day. I was also exercising entirely too much.

That's right. I said exercising *too much.*

I ate a very healthy diet, and even made an attempt to meditate daily. I was got up before dawn to go on long runs in the mountains. Then taught Yoga; plus, I had my own Yoga practice. On top of all this, I was raising a little girl.

One day I just hit a wall. Not literally, of course. But a figurative wall. And it figuratively knocked me right on my butt. And this time, I couldn't pick myself back up again.

I was flexible. I was thin. I was a vegetarian. I could turn myself into a pretzel, do a hundred push-ups without taking a break, and run 20 miles at a stretch without stopping. I looked like the picture of health to everyone who knew me. But inside, I was falling apart. I was taking excessive amounts of pills to manage my physical pain, and on top of that, I was depressed. I was falling apart at the seams from an invisible illness.

I was depressed because it seemed there was no way out of this cycle. To function, I would have to take pain pills for the rest of my life, and I knew that would eventually wreck my body. The clock was ticking, and I didn't know how long I had. I had also sacrificed my mental faculties for this. I knew it was only a matter of time before my mind and body would give up completely.

I was 29 when I was diagnosed with fibromyalgia. After all these years of what I thought was typical pain levels for sciatica and arthritis sufferers, I was finally informed (via the fibromyalgia diagnosis) it was actually much deeper than that.

I had always thought it seemed like I was dealing with a lot more pain than other people, even the ones who were also suffering from migraines, sciatica, digestive issues, and arthritis. I wondered if maybe my pain tolerance really was just low (like so many people had condescendingly told me). But considering the number of tattoos, piercings, and assorted other body modifications I had gritted my teeth through in my (somewhat reckless) youth, I knew my pain tolerance was pretty darn high!

What was crazy was that I helped numerous students deal with the symptoms of this very condition, so I already knew quite a bit about it and had been able to help others keep their fibromyalgia under control. And now here I was, finding out that I had been dealing with the same condition without knowing.

Because I had researched it so much already for the sake of my students, I had an action plan in mind as soon as I found out what it was. Since it is not well understood by doctors (in fact, no one even knew what it was until 1990), it is rather challenging to treat. Almost everything revolving around fibromyalgia involves speculation. But I didn't have to speculate. I had already seen what could help other people.

At least I finally had the justification that—yes—my invisible pain was very real.

I had been aware of the spiritual side of Yoga for quite a while at this point. I studied it daily and was putting everything I learned into practice as best I could. I tried to meditate every single day, but my mind was so exhausted that I had no focus, and meditation usually just left me feeling confused and disoriented.

I knew about the eight limbs of Yoga from all my reading and tried to put them into practice in my daily life. I had read *Autobiography of a Yogi* and knew that there were very deep levels of Yoga that one could achieve. I also knew this was not out of my reach; I just had to figure out how to apply myself.

I did my best to implement all the Ayurvedic principles I had learned as well. I carefully analyzed my own personal constitution and tried to alter my diet and lifestyle accordingly. Many people thought I was too radical with my lifestyle restrictions. There were so many foods I didn't eat; so many things I didn't do. But I knew I was never going to get better if I didn't put effort into it. I put all of my focus into being as disciplined as possible.

Eventually, though, it finally happened. It took until the age of 30. But I finally figured out how to turn my health around.

According to Ancient Chinese Medicine, disease starts in the gut. I had heard this many times throughout my life, but it hadn't clicked. It took my stomach rupturing, and my colon shutting down completely—which led to my body going into a septic state—for me to finally understand that disease certainly did start in the gut. I also knew that if that was true then *health* began in the gut as well.

This was the epiphany that changed everything for me.

The stomach pains I dealt with during and directly after my pregnancy had returned. Even though I wasn't eating gluten, and I was still on what I thought was a clean and healthy vegan diet, the pain had come back with a vengeance. The bloating was worse than ever.

The gas and cramping were excruciating and severe. And I was constipated *all the time.*

Also—although I hadn't made the correlation—the brain fog, dizziness, and confusion had gotten significantly worse as well. It never dawned on me that this was linked to my digestive issues.

Because I had been dealing with chronic pain my entire life, I had a pretty high tolerance. But this was the most painful experience I had encountered yet. And let me remind you—I had given birth to a 10-pound baby!

My time in the hospital "opened my eyes." It was time to reflect on everything I had been through; everything I had learned. And now, I was learning to apply it.

Initially, when I told the doctor the type of pain I was experiencing, she just shrugged and said, "You just need to eat more veggies."

I know my face fell when she said that to me. I just muttered, "But I'm vegan!" and then burst into tears.

That shut her up real quick.

The doctors and nurses were all shocked when I told them I was a vegetarian, on a high-fiber diet, and I didn't eat any sugar or grains. I also didn't drink alcohol, smoke, or eat any junk food at all.

So why didn't my digestive system work properly? I told them I knew it was from all the painkillers I had taken my whole life, but they said that was absurd.

A week in the hospital being tested, scanned, pumped, sliced open, poked, and prodded—and the only advice they sent me home with was: "Eat more veggies"!

Thank you so much for that, I thought. *I will be sure to refer your services to all my friends.*

I left the hospital with a new agenda. I decided to take a hiatus from teaching and made a deal with myself that I wasn't going to teach again until I had figured *myself* out.

I took another nutritional course based around the inner ecosystem of the digestive tract. This opened up a whole new world for me. I began to repair my digestive system using a ridiculously strict diet consisting almost entirely of vegetables. My new regime also included large amounts of probiotics, digestive enzymes, and my least favorite part; colon hydrotherapy. Within a week, my symptoms were lessening.

A week!

And I mean *all* my symptoms, not just the digestive problems. For the first time in my life, I felt good. My pain was lessening significantly by the day, and my mind was becoming clearer.

I continue this diet to this day. It isn't nearly as strict now, but I keep the basic principles in mind in everything I do. As my energy began to get better, my focus and mental clarity got better as well. I learned that by getting so much exercise—especially while taking excessive amounts of painkillers—I had damaged my blood pressure and my body's ability to adapt to stress or process nutrients.

I continued learning, took two more courses; one of them involved repairing the metabolism by adapting physical activities to your personal body type; the other one was focused solely on traditional Ayurveda and Yoga practices. This was something I had studied before but was now taking to a deeper level.

Eventually, thanks to an emergency room doctor in India (I told you, I travel a lot!), I was finally given the correct diagnosis. I had a systemic candida infection that had caused intestinal permeability (leaky gut) and chronic postural hypotension.

This may just sound like a lengthy and boring string of words to you, and it did to me at first as well, until I started looking into it and realized I had finally struck gold. These frustrating little details had been the basis of all my health issues for my entire life. One thing had led to another, the butterfly effect had taken place. Now here I was, 30 years old, in horrible pain, with zero ability to concentrate, and a body that functioned at the level of an 80-year-old woman.

I worked with an Ayurvedic doctor while I was in India to discover the root of my systemic candida infection. It all came down to a proper balance of acid/alkaline in the body. My pH levels. Once I started to adjust my body's pH levels toward a more alkaline state, my symptoms began to lessen. I did my best to avoid anything that could aggravate an acidic state in my body. It was sad because I had been a lover of spicy food my entire life.

But soon enough, I was getting migraines only once or twice a month, and I was able to keep my sciatica at bay altogether. The brain fog faded, and I actually *forgot* about my arthritis! For the first time in my life, I felt like a person. A real-life human being who could finally have conversations, stand up without feeling dizzy, bend over without crying, digest my food, and exercise without having a horrible crash afterward.

With all this newfound information (and by newfound, I mean thousands of years old!), I could hardly wait to share what I had learned with others. I knew this was going to change everything about the way I interacted with my students.

My entire life, I had wanted nothing more than to make a difference, and I knew this was going to be the way I would do it. I could *really* help people now. I had observed things in so many people over the years that made me wonder why some people could do things with such ease but others couldn't—no matter how much they challenged themselves.

With my physical health skyrocketing, my spiritual health increased as well.

I could go deeper in my meditations. My attitude shifted. I didn't get irritated or angered by things that would have bothered me in the past. My mood swings lessened, and eventually, stopped altogether. My patience increased. My compassion for others increased. My connection to the earth grew. I was filled with great love. My love continues to grow every day.

It's impossible to explain. But this inner peace I discovered transformed my entire personality. My wants and needs began to dissipate. I found myself happier with much less. And even when my pain did flare up again, it didn't send me into a state of depression like it used to. I learned to accept the pain for what it was: a learning experience. A chance to grow.

> Now I try to see everything as a chance to grow *spiritually*. When pain does flare up, I accept it with gratitude and set it aside. I don't let it control me anymore.

For this reason, I feel I can say I have overcome chronic pain. Even though sometimes the physical pain may come back, I don't allow it to affect my life negatively anymore. And, in all fairness, I don't even deal with much physical pain now anyway. After experiencing it as such an integral part of my life for almost 30 years, an occasional minor flare-up doesn't set me back the way it would have in the past.

But when I look back—all my pain was worth it because it gave me the tools I needed to help others. I suffered for a purpose because now I am using everything I learned from those experiences to change lives.

> If we see everything as a problem, we have to work harder. If we see everything as an opportunity to improve and apply it to our practice, we will have a very interesting and fulfilling life. It doesn't matter how long or short that life may be.

Gradually, I was able to take the bits and pieces of everything I learned, not just about Yoga, but Ayurveda, herbalism, Traditional Chinese Medicine, and Qigong, and put it to use. I was also able to combine my studies about the inner ecosystem, anatomy, detoxification, inflammation, metabolic reconditioning, and pH balancing, and form it into a system I could apply to others.

I watched my students transform as well. Even though I understood that each person had a unique body and situation, there were undoubtedly some general consistencies which applied to everyone. Through these experiences, I developed the four Mindful Movement Techniques™. By using these particular techniques, an individual can personalize their physical activities (especially Yoga sequences) to suit their specific needs.

The human body is genuinely *amazing* on so many levels. I have been fascinated since I first started learning about how it works in elementary school. It is also pretty fascinating, however, just how many things can go *wrong*.

We move about the earth in these extraordinary, high-functioning machines. These machines are—very literally—the vehicles for the soul. But, as B.K.S. Iyengar pointed out, "No one ever washes a rented car."

To poke at the "body as vehicle" metaphor a little further, let's make another comparison:

Consider a fuel system on a car; if you don't service the fuel filter, but you just keep putting gas in it and doing tune-ups, eventually the fuel filter picks up all that crap. If it has no way to get rid of it, then all the servicing and maintenance you do to the outside of the car won't matter, and the whole system will just start to fail.

If the filter is clogged up, it can't work as well, so it's going to start making the engine work harder. So the pistons have to use dirty fuel, and the fuel pump has to work harder.

Plus, other parts have to pick up its slack, which is going to wear them out, too, because they're not meant to work that hard. You're just going to start stressing overworking more parts throughout the car.

But if you get rid of that fuel system problem by fixing the filter and cleaning the area, then it will start to get better gas mileage and better longevity.

Everything is supposed to work together.

Now, remember your body is the car. And imagine your digestive tract is the fuel filter. The food you eat would be the gas, and the tune-ups would be occasional cleanses you do for your body to keep it running smoothly.

But none of those things you do for your body to keep it healthy work as well as they should because the deep inner problem hasn't been handled. But if we go in and service our inner fuel system, we will be able to get better mileage and longevity.

All the body systems really are supposed to work together. This type of metaphor explains why cleaning out the small intestine and getting your whole digestive tract to work correctly can actually remove many outer problems such as psoriasis or arthritis.

But how can you do it safely and efficiently? Keep reading.

ADOPTING MINDFULNESS

Now that I have told you about what I went through personally, and why I am so adamant to help others, I'm going to talk about *how*. We have talked about the *why*, and now it's time to talk about the *how*. This book is a big part of my how.

I feel it is important to note here that it is very difficult when it comes to Yoga to actually do it *wrong*. There are a lot of myths out there around Yoga (which I won't go into in this book, I spent enough time on that in *Yoga for YOU*). But the main thing is that many people believe if they start doing Yoga—but they aren't doing everything exactly the way they're supposed to be doing it—then it's not even worth doing.

This is not true. Because every body is entirely different, everyone is going to look different when they do these things—and do them a little bit differently. This is why I have discovered the Mindful Movement

Techniques™ are so incredibly beneficial for helping each body adapt.

There are, of course, some things that are not conducive to personal growth or overcoming pain when it comes to the Yoga postures, and it is correct that some things can be downright dangerous. But these are usually extreme cases. As we continue to practice, our bodies adapt, and we become more in tune with how everything is supposed to look and feel. Doing dangerous movements repeatedly will eventually damage the body, but usually—with a little mindfulness—we can make the adjustments and corrections necessary to avoid this.

This is what separates a beginner from an advanced Yoga practitioner. It's not flexibility, strength, or endurance. It is the practitioner's ability to be *mindful*. A genuinely mindful person is an advanced Yoga practitioner indeed.

No progress can be made if we can't learn to listen to our bodies. And our bodies have a lot to say to us. Our bodies can give us the guidelines we need to keep them fit and healthy. If you have been practicing Yoga for some time, and are not seeing any fruits of your actions, then you have not been mindful.

What is mindfulness?

In the simplest of terms it is just *paying attention.*

Instead of allowing our minds to wander, we remain rooted in the present moment. Instead of replaying the past or imagining the future, we let go of wanting things to be different—wanting more.

We are not aiming to control or suppress our thoughts. We simply pay attention to them as they arise —without judging them. Then we can just let them go without getting caught up in them or swept away.

This allows us to become the watcher or the observer of our thoughts and sensations. Which, in turn, allows us to consciously remove ourselves from the cycle of repeatedly playing out systematic ways of thinking and living that are not conducive to our evolution.

Absolutely anything we do in our daily life with attention and awareness can be considered a mindfulness practice then.

Why should we practice mindfulness?

Regarding the physical Yoga postures and the Mindful Movement sequences, mindfulness applies by being so present in our bodies that the outward sensations, thoughts, distractions, and fears don't affect what we do. This doesn't mean we completely zone out and ignore everything around us, but instead, we are simultaneously aware of everything.

In other words, we are *tuning in* instead of *tuning out*. *Zoning in* instead of *zoning out*. It doesn't mean we are lost in our own little world; it means we are fully present in the present moment. We are doing what we are doing and not bothered by what else is going on.

When we are mindful in our physical practice, we

become more aware of the sensations happening in the body. The more conscious we become, the more we will be able to notice and feel. When I first started practicing Yoga, I was blundering through the poses like a baby deer learning how to walk.

Someone watching me may have thought I was doing them fine, I had a dance background after all, so I made them look beautiful. But the difference between Yoga and dancing—for me—was that when I danced, I was focused entirely on how it *looked,* but when I practiced the Yoga postures, I became more and more aware of how they *felt.* And the effect they had on my body, mind, and spirit.

I have been practicing long enough now that I can literally feel the individual muscles inside my body. I can feel if my kneecap has shifted slightly to the right or if I need to activate my left hamstring. If I collapse my chest or my shoulders, I can feel it throughout my entire body, and I know when I unclench my toes and my jaw I can relax significantly deeper into whatever pose I'm doing.

Taking this several steps further, I can feel my heart beating inside my chest; I can feel the blood pulsing through my veins. I can feel my digestive tract pumping and the individual hairs on my skin.

To get to this point, I started with visualization techniques and, eventually, was able to feel the results. When I *visualize* more air filling up my lungs, I can physically *feel* it now. People can even see my torso expanding when they watch me.

When I *visualized* my digestive tract functioning at its optimal level, I was eventually able to *feel* it. I envisioned the arthritis and the inflammation dissipating from my joints and muscles. Now I can feel the effects of this as well.

I am especially sensitive to this during my Yoga practice, but it has become an everyday part of my life, too. It has taken a while, and I didn't even realize the progress was happening, but now that I look back, the journey has been incredible! I have made so much progress it's astonishing.

Just think, it all started with mindfulness.

And *anyone* can do this.

Mindfulness is no longer a hidden ancient concept. It is practiced by millions of people today. It is taught in schools, workplaces, and hospitals all over the world. Interest in mindfulness is exploding because of the incredible benefits.

First and foremost, it reduces stress and anxiety because it changes how the body responds to stress and unpleasant situations. It also reduces insomnia and addictive tendencies.

It reduces depression and increases our confidence and sense of well-being. It also reduces fatigue and increases energy on the mental and physical level. It even boosts our immune systems and assists the body in overcoming illness.

Mindfulness improves memory and increases focus and attention span. It helps with pain management. It improves relationships by developing our empathy and compassion.

Overall, this gives us the capacity to *choose* to be happy. It leaves us feeling fulfilled, peaceful, and whole. This is such an important concept—especially when it comes to something like a Yoga practice. The establishment of mindfulness will give us an attention and understanding of the breath and the body. This is crucial for catering our physical activities to our bodies' needs.

ACTION STEPS

Have you ever heard of the beginner's mind? It's an ancient concept with spiritual roots.

But it is still very relevant in our everyday life. The next time you sit down to a meal, imagine it is the first time you have ever tasted food.

This is usually pretty astonishing.

What is the texture like? The temperature? How would you describe the taste?

This can transform your entire experience of eating. You will find yourself enjoying the food more and really appreciate it.

The beauty of approaching everything with a beginner's mind is that it makes us more mindful of everything we see or do. And, with continued practice, this will bring special attention to areas of your being you ignored before.

Take a good look at your friend, spouse, child, or someone close to you. Have you ever noticed that little freckle above her eyelid? What about the way that little wisp of hair always sticks out? Maybe he smiles with one corner of his mouth before the other.

If you were looking at the person for the first time, these things would be clearer to you. Things we take for granted because we see them all the time.

Do you usually drink your morning cup of coffee mindlessly? Or do you notice the way it feels rolling over your tongue? Or sliding down the back of your throat?

One of my favorite ways I suggest you approach this technique is to use it the next time you step into the shower. Imagine this is your first shower ever.

What an experience! Hot water cascading over your skin. Steam opening up your pores. The smell of soap.

With some practice, this technique will begin to find its way into more of your activities. Being mindful of everything you do will begin to brighten every area of your life. You will find yourself becoming more appreciative and less distracted.

1: Finding Your Beginner's Mind

Even if this concept isn't new to you, you are going

to pretend like it is! That is the whole basis of *The Beginner's Mind.*

All you have to do today is take a shower.

Yes, a shower.

But this should be a *mindful* shower.

From the moment you turn on the water, pay attention to every sensation happening within you and around you. Feel the steam on your skin—the temperature in the room rising.

Is there a particular scent in the air?

Pay attention to every movement you make to get into that shower. Say to yourself, "I am stepping into the shower." "I am experiencing the sensation of the water on my skin."

Make a note of the temperature of the water. Exactly how it feels. Observe the sensation as the water hits your scalp.

Every little detail matters. Pay attention to every move you have to make to grab hold of your soap, shampoo, or washcloth. How does that feel against your skin? How does it smell? What thoughts and feelings does it evoke?

It doesn't matter if it is a long shower or a short shower; just pay attention to every sensation that occurs during the entire process. This will work just as well if you would prefer to take a bath. Just follow the same steps.

Continue paying attention as you dry yourself off—observing the feeling of the towel against your skin.

Continue to practice this mindfulness as you proceed with your routine that takes place after the shower.

Chances are, this is the most attention you have ever paid to your showering process. And this is a pretty amazing thing!

When you have finished, observe your body and ask yourself, "How do I feel now?"

You might feel a little different than usual. But observe the effects of operating with such mindful intentions.

2: THE MINDFUL MEAL

Every time you eat today, stop and take a moment to offer gratitude for what you are about to consume.

Try not to eat in a detached way. Sit down, turn off distractions, and *really pay attention* to your food!

Observe the color and texture—the temperature. Chew it slowly and swallow with intention.

Say to yourself, "I am chewing this rice," or "I am swallowing this carrot."

Then visualize your digestive tract and what it is doing. Imagine everything is being appropriately assimilated (especially if you tend to have digestive problems).

Remember, we all have a small ecosystem inside our digestive tracts that can only function at optimal levels when every part is working in a synergistic balance.

Do your best to keep yourself in balance by eating mindfully!

Try to remember to do this each time you eat.

3: Mindful Posture

Start by standing up straight in the middle of the room.

Close your eyes (if you have enough balance) and observe your posture.

Are you leaning forward or back? Or to one side?

Do you favor a particular foot?

Do you let your kneecaps collapse?

What about hunching your shoulders?

Try to balance everything. Be aware of what it feels like when you shift your center of gravity back and forth.

When you have found a sense of balance, take a deep breath in, tighten up all your muscles, and hold the breath for a few seconds while you tighten everything up.

Now, with a loud sigh, breathe out and relax the muscles you just tightened up. Try to remain balanced, though.

This is the type of posture you want to aim for all the time. Balanced and relaxed (but not slouching!).

You can do this anywhere, too. In line at the grocery store, in front of the bathroom mirror while you brush your teeth—wherever.

When your body learns that this posture is optimal

for functioning correctly, it will remember that, and you will begin to do it naturally.

These little mindfulness practices will eventually become second-nature if you continue to use them in your daily activities.

You will find that you are becoming more aware of everything. And when we become more aware, we can work more efficiently on becoming less attached to worldly activities and sensations.

So there we have it. Three helpful tips to include mindfulness in your daily life.

Now we are ready to move into the most important part of overcoming chronic pain.

SHIFTING MINDSET

A positive mindset shift is the single most important thing we can do to overcome chronic pain. It seems like such a little thing to so many, but it is absolutely pivotal when it comes to achieving overall health of the mind, body, and Spirit.

Our mindset is what can spring us forward in life to be successful and do the most incredible things. But it can also be what holds us back and keeps us where we are. Being deliriously happy or mind-numbingly miserable all depends entirely upon mindset.

Mindset is what sets apart the doers from the whiners. It is the most basic primordial instinct which can skyrocket people into success or set them back as the utmost failures. It is entirely up to us to choose happiness. To fully overcome chronic pain, we have to *choose* to do so. If we do not select this first and foremost, it will never really happen.

I can't stress this enough because this was the most prominent shift for me. In some ways, I was actually *comfortable* in my pain. I was so used to being miserable that I realized I wouldn't even know what to do with myself if I wasn't. *What would I talk about? Who would I complain to?*

I have seen this pattern in so many others as well. But the fact is, if you are comfortable in your pain, if you identify with it, if has become a part of who you are —you need to make that shift or you will never get better.

People who wallow in their pain on a daily basis and whine and complain or continuously ask the universe, "Why? Why is this happening to me? What did I do to deserve this?"—these are the people who don't get better because they aren't allowing themselves to. They get lost and caught up in the loop of negative thoughts.

I'm going to make another assumption here, and guess that you aren't one of those people now because you have picked up this book, and you are taking active steps to get better. But maybe you *were* one of those people, and perhaps it wasn't that long ago. I know I was.

But if you were—congratulations for taking the first steps in making that shift! Because deciding you want to get better is the most significant and challenging step you can take. It is, by far, the tallest hurdle you will overcome, and once you clear that hurdle, it will only get easier after that.

Now ask yourself this question: How tired *are* you of being sick?

Now I want you to read that again.

How tired are you of *being sick?*

Being sick has exhausted your body, mind, and spirit more than most of you realize. Or maybe you *do* realize it, and that is why you are so adamant to get better. But I need you to sit with that question for a little bit. Ask yourself, honestly, if you have put your chronic pain on the back burner of your life and just moved forward with all your activities without putting much thought into it. If this is the case, then it probably hasn't been at the forefront of your mind as the main thing you need to do to get better.

Until now.

So what has changed?

For so many of us, pain is the underlying monster in the closet that is always present in everything we do, think, or feel. But we keep locking it back in the closet so we can forget about it for certain stretches at a time. But this doesn't stop it from jumping out of the closet from time to time to scare the bejesus out of us and leave us traumatized over and over again.

For others, it is the giant pink elephant in the middle of the room. It is always there, and very obvious. That stupid elephant makes us miserable *all the time.* There is no way to ignore it, but we have become so accustomed to its presence we have trained ourselves—and our loved ones—to just move around it awkwardly as we go about our daily activities as best we can.

Whether your chronic pain is the monster in the closet or the pink elephant in the middle of the room; you are always aware of it on some level. It is always there. Or, if it's not, we are exceedingly grateful when we experience those pain-free minutes, hours, or days.

Chronic pain sufferers do have a benefit in the fact that gratitude is more prevalent when we *aren't* suffering. Most people don't even think about the fact they aren't hurting. They only think about pain when they *are* dealing with it. But most of the time they aren't. But when chronic pain is the norm, we are much more grateful when it isn't present.

I now I wake up every morning full of gratitude for the fact I can get out of bed without taking Vicodin. I offer up my gratitude to the universe and wish for it to go out into the world to improve the lives of everyone in it.

A very sad thing about chronic pain sufferers is the tendency to always have to lie. When someone asks you casually, "Hi, how are you?" in passing, the typical answer is, "I'm good, thanks, and you?" But someone dealing with chronic pain either has to lie and say they are doing well, or they launch into a string of negativity that nobody really wants to hear.

It is an inner battle. I know it was for me every time someone asked me how I was doing. And this happened several times a day. It was a tug of war for my ego between lying—which I didn't feel good about—or basically just complaining—which I didn't want to project on the other person. That long string of negativity affects everyone you throw it at.

Have you ever noticed how drained you feel around people who complain all the time? If somebody just whines and complains to you every time you see them, you want to be around them less. It's exhausting. I know I certainly don't want to *be* that person. It's like being an energetic vampire.

Getting to this point, however, isn't always easy. Most people tend to make a habit out of complaining. It can take a lot to shift a pattern or habit that has been part of our lives for so long. But there are some little things we can do to start.

Okay, so the first thing we need to do is completely get rid of the idea that anything is *bad* for us. Of course, we know in our heads that painkillers are not conducive to our overall well-being. However, it is entirely another thing to go around saying out loud, "These pain pills are destroying my stomach! I'm going to have to get half my stomach removed because of this! This is destroying my digestive tract and my well-being!" Constantly repeating these things to the universe makes them even more concrete in reality.

I am going to talk more about painkiller dependence in the next chapter, but for now I can tell you moving past the guilt surrounding me was the number one hardest thing for me to get past. Every time the pain would get so overwhelming I would have to take a pain pill—even if it was just ibuprofen—I would be so wrought with guilt it would send me into a state of depression.

So maybe I wasn't feeling the pain *physically* for a few hours, but I was certainly feeling it *emotionally*. Sometimes it's a matter of sorting out your priorities. In the beginning, the pain pills are still going to be a part of your journey. We need to just accept that that's okay and move forward. The dependency on pain pills will eventually dissipate on its own. But trying to force it is only going to add more stress to an already delicate situation.

People would always refer to me as a delicate flower. But I prefer to think of myself as more of a fragile cactus. I have toughened myself up, but it doesn't mean I'm going to go out and do anything stupid that could harm me in the long run.

What if your primary *why* for wanting to overcome chronic pain is to be able to spend more time with your children and be more involved in their lives; but in order to go to your daughter's dance recital this evening, you need to take a painkiller? Then feeling guilty about it isn't going to help you.

As you swallow the pill, say to yourself, "It is doing my body only good, and it is helping me." Take the painkiller with intention, and go enjoy your daughter's dance recital. Once again, it's a matter of priorities.

If you are lying at home sick in bed and utterly

miserable in your pain, you will only be twice as miserable because not only are you dealing with physical hurt because you didn't take the pill, but you are missing your daughter's dance recital anyway. If that painkiller will take the pain away for a few hours, long enough for you to go support your child and be there for her and have that memory, and that is worth it to you—because you have made it your priority—then do it! And don't allow the guilt to creep in. Remember you would feel significantly more guilt for *not being there.*

> Tell yourself you are already perfect because you truly are. The situation will improve if you believe it will.

The next step, and remember these are baby steps—little changes that create a ripple effect for a big outcome—is to start shifting into the mindset of *feeling great.*

I started with repeating regularly, "I feel great."

It was a simple little affirmation that became my mantra. This is actually a concept taught in Yoga, but at the time, I hadn't even made the connection.

A mantra is a repeated series of sounds and words to form a prayer. When it is repeated over and over (usually 108 times which is the number of beads on a mala) these words build power. And remember, words have *tremendous* power! The vibration of a word you put out into the world shifts the vibration of everything around you.

That is why I get so uncomfortable when someone says the F-word around me. Especially *at* me. It's this vibrational punch in the face you are putting out into the world whether you realize it or not. After practicing mindfulness for so long, we tend to become even more empathic and can feel things like this to the utmost degree.

On the other end of the spectrum, however, we can positively shift the vibration by putting positive words out into the world. Sanskrit (which is the ancient language the *Yoga Sutras* were initially written in, as well as the language in which most prayers and mantras are chanted in India), is still alive today because it is so vibrationally powerful.

The combination of sounds in the letters and words in Sanskrit are divinely inspired and built to create a positive vibrational ripple more than any other series of sounds. This is why chanting *Om*—the primordial sound of the universe—is so healing. This can even be compared to Christianity in the Bible, where it says:

"In the beginning was the Word, and the Word was with God, and the Word was God."

— JOHN 1:1

Many believe this *Word* can be compared to the sacred sound of *Om.* Which, in the Christian tradition, translates to *Amen*: a holy seal with the meaning, *so be it,* that has so much healing power.

No matter what religion you abide by, if any at all, there is no denying that words have power. Children who continuously hear they are stupid end up believing it. And unfortunately, usually become that.

So to entirely shift the mindset, we have to start by directing our energy in a positive and healing way. "I feel great," is what I started with, and it worked for me very well. I tried to remember to do it occasionally, but soon I was chanting it silently in my head all the time. Now I have a mantra I chant daily in Sanskrit which was given to me by my *guru* (spiritual teacher). But even from time to time nowadays, I remind myself that *I feel great!* I am healthy, happy, and grateful to be alive!

Maybe you have heard that forcing yourself to smile all the time will eventually make you happy? It's the same concept. Your brain reacts to these physical things on an emotional level. You can actually reprogram your mind and body to feel better by doing these types of activities.

So, every morning, as soon as you wake up, even if you are stiff, achy, or writhing in pain, say to yourself, "I feel great." It might feel awkward and forced at first, but eventually, it will become more comfortable. And then one day it will feel natural.

Whenever you think about it, say to yourself, "I feel great." For even more power, look at yourself in the mirror, make eye contact with your reflection, and repeatedly say out loud, "I feel great."

This leads me to the necessity of applying proper verbiage. The way we word things can make a big difference in the outcome. It's all a matter of assessing where we are, where we want to be, and what we are trying to do. Our words play a big part in this. So try to pay attention or be mindful of the words you use throughout the day.

How much time do you spend complaining or feeling sorry for yourself? Naturally, we all slip up sometimes; I still do this, of course. But almost every time a complaint slips out of my mouth, I catch myself faster and faster. The first thing I do, if I accidentally make a negative comment about something, is I immediately try to follow it up with something positive. It's kind of like hitting the CANCEL button on the universe's dashboard.

The universe can hear what you put out there. So if everything that comes out of our mouth is negative, the universe is just going to give us a whole lot more of that: negativity. If everything we say reinforces the concept that we are in pain and we are suffering, it just further secures us into the loop of endless pain and suffering.

So I try to observe my words now. I do my best to speak with intention. If someone asks me how I'm doing, I focus on the positive. I am careful to pay attention to what I say, and if you want to get better, you should, too.

So just remember, in order to get better, we need to forget about *trying*. Let's throw that completely out of our vocabularies. Let's focus on *doing*. We do not *try*, we *do!*

In the wise words of Yoda:

"Do or do not. There is no try."

That little wrinkly green guy gave me a lot to think about in my lifetime!

ARE YOU DEPENDENT ON PAINKILLERS?

As I mentioned in the previous chapter, I want to talk more about painkiller dependence and why this is such a hot topic for chronic pain sufferers. Chances are, if you suffer from chronic pain, you have some experience with prescription and nonprescription pain medications. I already told you about some of my issues with it, but this is so important I will now revisit it.

PAINKILLER DEPENDENCY SHAME

Painkiller dependency can be a touchy subject, but it is a BIG topic for chronic pain sufferers!

There is probably a good chunk of you out there who are reading this right now, who are entirely dependent on painkillers. Absolutely no judgment if you are because I've been there. There was a very big portion of my life I couldn't even get out of bed in the morning without them.

Like I said earlier, I went through all kinds of things. I was prescribed Vicodin from a ridiculously young age. So I understand—I have been taking heavy amounts of painkillers my entire life. It was never for any kind of addiction reasons. Or because I wanted to get high off of them.

It was because I was in *freaking pain,* and it was the only way I could actually function on a human level.

PILLS ONLY HELP UNTIL THEY HURT

But the problem was eventually the painkillers started making me *not* feel good anymore. They started giving me brain fog and dizziness, and I just wasn't myself anymore. But I was in so much pain if I didn't take them, I thought that was my only choice.

I was taking copious amounts because I was in pain *all the time* and I just wanted to be normal.

> Wanting to be normal is the main reason for painkiller dependency with chronic pain sufferers.

QUITTING "COLD TURKEY"

When I started having severe problems with my digestive tract, I knew this was because of all the painkillers I was taking. So I started weaning myself off of them at one point, but then I decided they were so bad for me I would go cold turkey.

That was the *worst* idea ever! So if you're thinking about just ending your painkiller usage abruptly, I really don't recommend that because of the horrible withdrawals. And honestly, my body went into shock, so I really don't recommend that for *anyone*. It is true that everyone is different, but why take the chance?

When I first published a blog post about this, I got tons of comments from people stating they went off painkillers cold turkey with no issues. Well, good for them. That's just fine and dandy, but that was *not* the case for me or *anyone* I know!

BABY STEPS

The best things we can start to do is to neutralize the effect the painkillers have on our bodies—especially our stomachs, livers, and kidneys—are little physical things, like just to take food with the painkillers. Don't take the stuff on an empty stomach because you really need to have something protective in your stomach to actually combat the effects the pills have.

A helpful tip is take a tablespoon of coconut oil

every time you take a pain pill. This coats your entire digestive tract and neutralizes the negative effects of the pill.

Another thing I HIGHLY recommend—and this is definitely a little more esoteric—is pay attention to your mindset. When you take that pill, give thanks for what it's doing to actually help your body. Tell yourself that you're *healing.*

This isn't hurting your body! Say, "This is good for me and it's only going to *do* good for me."

SO IN WITH THE GOOD, OUT WITH THE BAD!

Just visualize that your body is processing only the parts of that pill that are going to help it not have pain, and it's going to expel all the toxins and any sort of negative effects it could have on the rest of the body. Just keep telling yourself that—really visualize it, and you have to really believe it. When you do this, it really does make a big difference over the long run.

And eventually, little by little, as we go through these steps . . . our need for the painkillers will lessen.

AS THE BODY GETS CLEANER, IT PROCESSES THINGS BETTER

It expels all the bad stuff more efficiently. We actually start to feel less pain. Then we don't need the painkillers as often. Slowly but surely.

For me, it took about 15 years of slowly weaning

myself off of the pain pills before I didn't need them anymore. A lot of my clients have had *way* faster results —and good for them! But for me, it was a long process. Though I can't even begin to describe to you how much better I feel now that I don't need them as often.

Overcoming painkiller dependency doesn't necessarily mean we can get off painkillers for the rest of our lives (although some really are!). Every once in awhile, some of us might still need to reach for that little orange bottle from time to time—even if it's just a Tylenol or something—but just know that if you do, *it's okay.*

LETTING GO OF GUILT

So you know sometimes it is okay. The main thing is just not having guilt. Because there's even a new disorder that they've named recently, called Orthorexia Nervosa. It's been coming about—especially in modern days, with all these fad diets out there—it's basically a disorder that we are *giving ourselves.*

Another simple term for this is *Food Guilt*—this is a very real condition and it is running rampant in many cultures (especially the West). Because there are so many people feeling so much guilt for eating things they know are bad for them, it's actually causing *even more* distress and digestive problems in their bodies.

And not just physical. There are other mental issues that come along with these disorders as well.

It is definitely something to think about if you are

on a vegan diet but you spend all of your time dreaming about cheeseburgers. Then you go out and eat a cheeseburger and feel so guilty about it, it does even more damage to your body than it would have if you hadn't had that guilt in the first place.

Just saying.

The same thing goes with painkillers. If you're taking a painkiller, and the whole time it's going down through your system, you're thinking, *this is so bad for me. I shouldn't have done this. I'm such a failure. I'm weak....* It will have a lot worse effects on your body.

JUST GIVE THANKS

So, just remember to take medications with gratitude and be gentle on yourself. You are strong! You are a warrior! Overcoming painkiller dependency takes time. The fact that you're reading this means you've taken a step to actually overcome this pain. And that's a *huge* deal! So you are *amazing*. Give yourself a pat on the back. You know you are awesome. And so do I.

Just remember *no guilt, no guilt,* NO GUILT! You are perfect the way you are!

Even if you do not always feel that way.

That doesn't mean you shouldn't have the motivation to heal. But you also need to accept where you are so that you can move forward.

Guilt will only cause *emotional chronic pain*. Which I will go into next.

EMOTIONAL CHRONIC PAIN

Here is a detail I would like to touch on. The depths of this subject cannot be covered in this book, but I must express the common link between physical and emotional chronic pain.

Many of us who have been suffering from chronic pain for our entire lives have also suffered from deep-seated emotional or even physical abuse. So many students I work with have dealt with severe abuse and trauma in childhood which radiated into their adult lives and expressed itself as chronic physical pain.

When we deal with traumatizing life events, especially in our youth, we internalize these experiences because our young minds don't know how to process them yet.

If we are lucky, we can seek help in the future and handle them as needed. But for many of us, we internalize these things and forget they are there. Or we try to ignore them. Then they come forward in adolescence and adulthood as chronic emotional and physical problems. This is something to think about if you have been dealing with chronic pain for a significant portion of your life.

Take a look deep inside yourself. Are there deep-seated emotional issues from your past that you haven't adequately addressed? I know this was certainly the case for me. One of my students even told me that after she assessed this, she realized her most prominent points of physical pain on her body were the areas her mother used to hit her when she was a child. This is extremely common for children who have suffered abuse.

It is also vital that we take a look at our patterns throughout our lives as well. If we have suffered abuse as a child, it is common to unconsciously seek out abusive situations into our adulthood, too. It can go many ways, but the two most common paths are for the abused child to fully embody the victim role into adulthood, or they become the abuser.

But this is a cycle we do not have to succumb to. If we can take an in-depth look at these issues, perhaps seek outside psychological help, and really address these things to the point we can actually let them go; we may finally have the tools to eradicate chronic pain in our lives for good.

The vicious chronic pain cycle has so many faces. Many of us are not just suffering from *physical* pain. But it comes full circle, and we end up suffering from *emotional pain* about being in pain! We end up conditioned to think we are weak, inadequate, or useless because we are suffering.

If we feel like a burden on our friends and family, this causes the emotional pain to exacerbate the physical pain and vice versa. But if we can assess this, acknowledge it, and then make a conscious effort to break this cycle, we can truly step into the healing mindset.

For those of you this applies to—and you know who you are—this is your most important next step.

ACTION STEPS

I am going to share with you some suggested visualizations that have helped many of my students and me. Some of them can be a little bit uncomfortable to do, and if it's too scary, don't do it at first.

But eventually, I really feel all these visualizations are super important to ultimately overcome chronic pain. So just remember that and approach them with an open mind.

VISUALIZATION #1 - *OFFER YOUR PAIN TO THE UNIVERSE for recycling.*

This has been a very helpful visualization for me, and I still use it to this day. This is the technique that helped me move past my feelings of hopelessness and worthlessness that revolved around my chronic pain.

My pain was so severe that I couldn't even take care of myself properly, let alone my child when I finally became a mother. I felt entirely dependent on other people and painkillers. This left me feeling utterly useless because I felt like I'd never be able to do anything on my own.

On top of all that, I thought I was suffering pointlessly. There was absolutely no purpose for this pain.

But then I met a Buddhist monk who shared something with me that changed everything: Energetically, we can offer our pain to the universe for recycling. We can set an intention when we are suffering that we are putting it out into the world to actually alleviate some of the sufferings of others—making a universal impact.

If you are a parent, and you have ever sat with your sick child, you know just how much you wish you could take that child's pain away. But what if you could? What if, by suffering, you focus your attention so pointedly on removing the sufferings of others it actually gives your pain a purpose?

This creates a vast transformation when applied to painful situations. This concept goes way back with many different religious roots. According to the Christian tradition, Christ died on the cross to atone for all of our sins.

The Buddhist and Hindu religions openly accept the fact that we can make things better by putting positive energy out there into the rest of the world to raise the vibration. So by suffering with intention, we can actually *vibrationally lessen the sufferings of others on a global level.*

Every little bit counts. Now, every time I feel pain, I put my hands on the ground next to me and visualize feeding my pain back into the earth for recycling back out into the world. I envision my suffering actually lessening the sufferings of others because I am consciously taking on and burning up their negative karma.

This gives me tremendous peace. I can't even describe to you the amount of comfort this has given me over the years and still does to this day. It's hard to fully understand unless you try it. So out of all the chronic pain visualizations I have studied, this one has been by far the most effective for me (and many people I know as well).

VISUALIZATION #2 - *IMAGINE THE WORST-CASE SCENARIO.*

This one can be a tough one. And it's actually so scary and uncomfortable for some people they can't even do it right away. But eventually, as you become more comfortable with these practices, the fear will begin to dissipate, and eventually, so will the pain. This particular method helped me cut down on my painkiller usage.

One day I had a terrible migraine. As I was reaching for the bottle of pills, I had a thought. *What if I didn't take them? What would happen? What is the absolute worst thing that would happen?*

The pain would get worse. My head would pound. The throbbing would get overwhelming and eventually turn my stomach, and I'd be vomiting. After that, I'd be dizzy and sick, and I wouldn't be able to see clearly. I would be in *so much pain.*

But then what? I'm in pain. So what? What do I do with that pain? Would I just continue to run from it?

We all tend to run from pain. It's fundamental human nature: Seek pleasure. Avoid pain. Makes perfect sense. But why do we do this? What makes pleasure so wonderful and pain so terrible? What if we could just accept our pain and move on?

Now I'm not saying I can walk around like a serene little fairy princess when I have a pounding migraine and not let it bother me in the slightest. No, it's freaking terrible. There is no denying that. But another ancient proverb states, "Pain is mandatory. Suffering is optional." And that is so true.

As I imagined dealing with the migraine at its absolute worst, a sense of peace began to wash over me. *I* wasn't the one suffering, and I wouldn't *be* the one suffering. My *body* would be suffering. But my body isn't *me.*

When we are sick, we have to remember that it's not actually that *we* are sick. Our *bodies* are sick. And that is something totally different. This level of non-attachment changes everything for a chronic pain sufferer. The more I continue to do this visualization of the worst-case scenario with my pain (and I did it with more than just my migraines; I did it with all of my issues), the less fear I experience around that pain.

Eventually, I decided to try and see what would actually happen. So the next time I got a migraine, I didn't take any painkillers. I can't really say I handled it all that well. But the point was, I handled it.

The migraine lasted for four days. Four days of excruciating agony. But as the pain got worse and worse, eventually, it came to a point where I realized that nothing could really hurt me. My soul was absolutely invincible, and this was incredibly freeing.

Now, I'm not saying I always avoid painkillers completely when I feel a migraine coming on. At that particular time, I just happened to be able to take those four days to myself and try to recover. And it actually took several days after the migraine ended for me to recover fully. But I don't always have that kind of time on my hands.

Once again, it's all about priorities. Sometimes I know I need to choose spending time with my daughter or getting my work done as my number one priority. But the point is, I did it. I didn't die. My soul is fine. And now I have a new sense of freedom and of being indestructible.

. . .

Visualization #3 - *Past, present, and future self.*

The third one I want to share with you is the visualization of where we are now and where we want to be. My mentor calls this the *Crystal Ball Meditation*. It is an extremely powerful manifesting technique which can be used for anything, such as an ideal relationship or financial abundance.

Sit in a comfortable seated position and assess yourself; your physical body, your state of mind, and your current spiritual state. Notice all the little things in your body; any places of tension, any points of pain.

Notice your postural alignment and just really pay attention to how you are feeling. If you have any extreme discomfort or pain, just imagine you are breathing into those areas and try to let it go. Sometimes this is more of an intention than an *actual* letting go.

Now hold your hands out in front of you as if you're holding a giant crystal ball. I now have an actual crystal ball made out of solid rose quartz that my daughter gave me as a gift when she saw me doing this visualization every morning. This has made the visualization even more powerful and personal for me, but make sure if you do choose to use a real crystal ball, it is a type of crystal that resonates strongly with your personality and constitution.

Inside the crystal ball, visualize yourself as you wish to be. Picture yourself at the place you want to get yourself to; physically, mentally, and spiritually. How does your skin look? Your hair? Your weight? Your posture? How does it look? Where are you? What is around you?

How do you ideally see yourself in the future? And where?

Now go a little deeper. How do you *feel?* Remember this is the ideal version of you. What is the temperature of your skin? How does your body feel? What about your mind? Are you thinking clearly and feeling good?

Now go another level deeper. Where are you *spiritually?* Are you completely content with who you are and how your life is? This is *your* visualization, so do whatever it takes to get to the ideal place you want to be. Does this mean full-blown enlightenment? Christ-consciousness? Nirvana? Samadhi?

Imagine you are completely overflowing with love and compassion. Your whole body is now filling with divine white light that is emanating out of you and into the world around you, raising the vibration on a global level. Your hands might even be vibrating at this point. *Really feel it.*

Now, mentally take that glowing crystal ball full of all of your ideals and place it somewhere in a safe place in your past. For me, this is the gazebo that used to be in my parents' backyard of my childhood home. There were beautiful plants and trees and a garden all around it, and it was my favorite place in the world. This is where I place my crystal ball, and then I watch as my inner child steps into the scene and sits down in a meditative position with the crystal ball.

Now bring your attention back to your hands, and start this visualization all over again. It can be a little bit faster this time, but once again, picture your ideal self—your best version of you—inside this crystal ball.

Once again filling up with light, mentally pick up the crystal and place it in a safe location in your future. This part can be a little bit harder to picture because you aren't there yet.

I visualize my distant future and exactly where I want to be at a certain point in time. It is a place I go in India that I intend to return to over and over again throughout my life. But if you are still very uncertain, use a place in your near future. It can even be in your own home.

Once you set it down, visualize your future self sitting with it. The future version of yourself that is completely healed. The exact version you wish to be.

Return your attention now to where you're sitting. Now there are three versions of you meditating together. Your past, present, and future. All three of you are meditating on the same thing—your ideal self. The best version of you.

While you sit here, envision the crystal balls beginning to expand, grow, and put out tremendous light. This light continues to travel outward until it is covering the entire Earth and pulsating out into the universe.

Your past and your future are now linked to each other, and your present is right there in the middle, amidst this white light. As the light continues to get stronger and continues to expand, visualize it dissolving into a dazzling, glitter-like substance and shooting outward into the universe.

THESE THREE MEDITATIONS/VISUALIZATIONS ARE THE most powerful and effective tools I have to offer you to help you shift your mindset.

Now it's time to get a little more physical.

GETTING TO KNOW YOU

Now let me backtrack a little. I decided to start with the most important aspects, but now I'm going to return to the initial things that are so important for laying a framework essential to healing. Let's imagine your mindset has already shifted and you have become one with your pain to the extent that nothing bothers you anymore. Wouldn't that just be lovely? And while I agree, that would be absolutely divine; we still have to pay attention to our physical bodies as well.

Sadly, I have met many spiritual practitioners, and even people who consider themselves enlightened, who pay absolutely no attention to their physical bodies.

Now, I certainly agree that healing takes place first in the mind, but that doesn't mean we should ignore the body! Sure, there are actual legitimate enlightened masters out there who don't care about their bodies at all. They care only about their oneness with God. But unless you are a living Buddha—which I know *I'm* not—it's pretty darn important to pay attention to these meat-suits carrying us around!

Remember the rented car metaphor? Let's talk about that again.

Sure, these bodies may be temporary, but we still want them in pristine condition so they can function their best to serve us while we have them. So it takes a lot more than just washing the rented car, we have to service the fuel filter, the engine, the internal computer—everything! And if we are dealing with chronic pain, that means something has gone awry, and we need to figure out the root of the problem. We need to go into the inner workings of our vehicles and service all of it. From the inside out.

The mind-body-spirit synergy, trilogy, Trimurti, sacred triangle—whatever you want to call it—has been studied for generations and for good reason. The three aspects relate to each other on multiple levels.

This is the part where we have to assess our physical and mental state. This took me the longest, by far, out of everything I learned—figuring out my body and mind.

For most people, it is essential to start with the mind, then we have to work on correcting imbalances in the physical body. This is where practices such as Ayurveda come in handy. I'm going to get into the fundamentals of Ayurveda in a moment, but first, I would like to encourage you to mosey on over to the resource section at the back of this book. There you will find references to books and websites that will help you discover your primary Ayurvedic constitution.

This is no substitute for a personalized consultation, but it will help give you a better idea of where to start. Then these next Ayurvedic principles you are about to read over will make more sense to you, and you can apply the following theories and methods a little more accurately to your own personalized and unique situation.

Determining which category (or categories) you fall into can really help point you in the right direction with the laser-sharp focus you need.

Like I have said, every *body* is different, so everyone has different needs. I'm not going to go into excessive detail here because it would be impossible to generalize everything without doing a personalized consultation where we break down the fundamentals and go deep into what is right for each individual's constitution.

AYURVEDA IN A NUTSHELL

Ayurveda is considered to be Yoga's sister science and is approximately five thousand years old. It is the ancient healing tradition of India and Nepal. Today it is a government-supported, health care system that is widely accepted, and whose methods are often practiced in conjunction with those of other modern medicine.

The major difference between Ayurvedic medicine and Western medicine, especially, is that Western medicine generally treats only the symptoms of disease, while Ayurveda treats the whole person. If you can find the source of the disease, the symptoms will be eliminated.

This, of course, takes time and patience and an understanding of the principles. You don't go to an Ayurvedic doctor for a pill to make your symptoms go away. You go to an Ayurvedic doctor with an open mind and an understanding that you will have to do what the doctor says and make changes in your life to allow yourself to heal.

Ayurveda asserts that true healing must occur on all levels of the being: physical, emotional, mental, and spiritual. It is not a substitute for Western medicine or a medical diagnosis but can work in conjunction accordingly.

Ayurveda works with methods of prevention and treatment, and common ways include Yoga practices, diet, internal cleansing, lifestyle adjustments, and individualized herbal formulations.

All of life contains a mixture of certain elements. And, in which, individual life-forms can be functionally grouped into three *doshas*—or constitutions. These are **Vata**, **Pitta**, and **Kapha**.

All three of these aspects exist in every living thing. But the ratio of these elements varies from one individual to another. This forms what is called a *Prakriti*, or individual constitution. This is the doctrine of the *Tridosha*, which Ayurvedic theory is based upon.

Vata: Known as the king of the doshas.

This element is a coordinated functioning of air and space. It manifests in the functioning of the nervous system, movement, cognition, and speech. Its nature is light, spacious, expansive, cold, dry, rough, mobile, changeable, and empty.

When balanced, it manifests as:

- Enthusiasm
- Curiosity
- Liveliness
- Creativity
- Empathy
- Sensitivity
- Intuition

In excess, it manifests as:

- Dry skin
- Lack of lubrication in the spine and joints
- Chronic chilliness
- Low blood pressure
- Heart palpitations
- Excessive urination
- Insomnia
- Hyperactivity
- Emaciation
- Chronic fatigue
- Irregular sleep/digestion/energy level
- Mental or nervous disorders such as panic or anxiety attacks
- Depression
- Mood swings
- Sensitivity
- Inability to concentrate

- Lack of groundedness

In general, Vata excess can be treated by warming, calming, and lubricating.

PITTA: CORRESPONDS TO FIRE. AND IN SOME SCHOOLS OF Ayurveda, it corresponds to water, also.

Present in the body's metabolic processes. Its nature is hot, sharp, penetrating, oily, and intense.

When balanced, it creates:

- Sharp intellect
- Logical processes
- Courage
- Inspiration
- Confidence
- Thirst for knowledge
- Ambition

In excess, it can be expressed as:

- Acne or skin rashes
- Inflammation
- Peptic ulcers
- Irritable Bowel Syndrome
- Stress
- Hypertension
- Heart attacks

- Hyperthyroid problems
- Competitiveness
- Anger
- Short temper
- Irritability
- Frustration
- Excessive drive for achievement
- Tendencies to manipulate, criticize, and control others
- Overly quick to react
- Aggressiveness
- Overheating

It can be neutralized by cooling and calming.

KAPHA: LINKS DIRECTLY TO EARTH AND WATER.

This element tends to be solid, heavy, cool, wet, stable, receptive, and inert.

When balanced, it creates:

- Good humor
- Calmness
- Gratitude
- Commitment and responsibility
- Caring for the physical needs of others
- Patience
- A feeling of fulfillment

When imbalanced, it manifests as:

- Obesity
- Diabetes
- Clinical depression
- Chronic mucous
- Asthma
- Tumors
- Edema
- Repression of emotions
- Greed
- Heaviness
- Dullness
- Lack of motivation
- Denial
- Sluggish metabolism
- Excessive sleep
- Excess weight
- Laziness

When provoked, it can be treated by warming, drying, and stimulating.

When attempting to treat any of these imbalances, it is important to remember that proper digestion is the root of good health.

All three of the doshas can be treated from the gut. It

is important to pay attention to cravings as well. They tend to represent an attempt by the body and mind to communicate their needs to each other and to balance themselves. When you are more balanced, you tend to crave tastes and flavors that will decrease the most predominant dosha. However, this requires an attunement with your body. Usually, this type of receptiveness can only be applied with time.

Typically, symptoms such as gas, burping, constipation, pain, or diarrhea, are examples of the body's attempt to communicate that it cannot digest or assimilate the substances that we are putting into it.

This means that it will not be able to separate what is good for the body from what needs to be excreted. This leads to the absorption of toxins. If you persist in forcing it to take in these indigestible substances, the long-term absorption of toxins may lead to various symptoms, such as chronic fatigue, lack of motivation, depression, allergies, arthritis, autoimmune disorders, and cancer.

Regarding chronic pain, it is important to note where the pain actually resides in the body. This can be an indicator of where it is coming from. Every source of chronic pain is coming from one of the three doshas or some sort of combination.

This is why I have my students fill out so many assessments and questionnaires even before my initial consultation with them. When we can determine our constitution, therefore, our tendencies toward imbalances, it can craft a clear path to the answer of how to reverse it. I build a "roadmap" with my students so that we can figure out which path they took, and from where, and then figure out how to back up enough to find the correct path to healing.

I could write hundreds of books full of new information about Ayurveda, and many have. I highly recommend delving into the subject more if you are really serious about being able to heal yourself. In order to achieve a balanced state, however, the focus in this book is how it relates specifically to *chronic pain*.

ACID VS ALKALINE

There is a lot of hype out there right now about the importance of an *alkaline diet*. You can buy expensive bottles of alkaline water in the health food stores and spend hundreds, if not thousands, every month on smoothie mixes and supplements to alkalize your body. But, in all honesty, none of this is necessary. In fact, if your body is so toxic and acidic to the point it can't even properly absorb these nutrients, all these expensive alkalizing "miracle-formulas" are completely pointless!

When the body is in an overly acidic state, everything just goes haywire. Even the most alkaline bodies are always going back and forth between a state of acid and alkaline. This varies from the part of your body to the time of day.

When you wake up first thing in the morning, especially if you are sleep-deprived, you tend to be more acidic. This is why so many of us wake up with halitosis (morning breath). It is because the body goes into an acidic state while we sleep. That disgusting smell that could strip paint which is emanating from our mouths when we wake up is actually coming from the *gut.*

When the digestive system is acidic, it is moving all the way up through the entire digestive tract and coming out of the mouth. People who eat a lot of sweets at night or who eat right before bed tend to wake up significantly more acidic than those who avoid food a few hours before laying down. Also, if we wake up sleep-deprived, we are acidic. Period.

The digestive system is a finely tuned and very organized hard-working machine. Just like the rest of the body. But I find it particularly fascinating. The problem is, it slows way down at night while we sleep. So as I said earlier, if we put a bunch of food in the stomach and then lay down, all the stomach acid the body produces to digest this food goes to the side of the stomach and just kind of sits there.

The body has to work a lot harder to push food through the digestive tract when we are lying down. But the problem is, when we are sleeping, the body is going into 'rest and recuperation' mode. Not 'hard-working digestion' mode. So the food just sits there in its own juices—and rots.

Other things that tend to make the body extremely acidic are, obviously, acidic foods. But these might not be what you think they are. Acidic foods are things like meat, eggs, cheese, sugars, and even nuts. There are acidic fruits, such as tomatoes and citrus, which most people are familiar with because they are told by doctors not to eat these things if they deal with ulcers or heartburn. But these fruits are technically the least of our worries.

Processed foods are by far the worst contenders here. This is about as acidic as you can get. And if you want to make your body as unbalanced as possible, go out and eat a bunch of processed food.

Now I'm not a big believer in telling you all the things you *shouldn't* eat. I am, however, a believer in suggesting the things you *should* eat. You probably know you shouldn't be eating a Big Mac, but let's be honest, if you choose to eat one, you're going to do it whether I tell you it's good or bad for you. So I will spare you. Let's focus on the good things.

Eating alkalizing foods will alkalize your body overall. But once again, I must reiterate it is vastly important to recondition the body to accept these nutrients to begin with. I know a lot of people who tried to go on a raw vegan diet (myself included) and felt fantastic for the first few months but then couldn't figure out why they got so sick.

It wasn't because the raw vegan diet was unhealthy, it was because our bodies were so toxic and sick that we weren't even able to process these good things we were putting in them. The digestive system went into shock, and everything went haywire. Instead of absorbing and processing the nutrients, the immune system went into overdrive and filled up with stomach acid and gas. This causes the painful cramping and bloating I was so familiar with for so long.

Thankfully, there are many ways to combat this. And it isn't even that difficult. I will go into the list of foods that can help with this process at the end of this chapter.

Let's start with the simplest thing we can do: hot water.

Yep. Hot water. That's it.

If you were to take only one thing out of this entire book to implement into your life (after mindset), I recommend it be the hot water. One to three cups of hot water every morning and at least one cup every evening before bed. And then as many as you can stand throughout the day. Just hot water. Nothing else added.

The reason this is so helpful and alkalizing is that the hot water nourishes the colon. Because it is warmer than your body, it is slowly absorbed all the way down from the moment it enters the body. It goes all the way through the digestive tract and hydrates the entire thing, whereas cold water shocks the system, shoots straight through your kidneys—causing stress on them—and then to your bladder. So you have to pee a lot, but you still aren't hydrated.

Perhaps, if you had a pristinely functioning, top-notch system, you would be able to drink cold water all the time and be fine, but chances are, if you're reading this book, then your system is not functioning top-notch. So drink the dang hot water!

Another important thing to note here is that a toxic body doesn't respond as well to herbs and supplements, or any natural healing method. I now understand this is why, in my youth, when I was trying to go completely natural, and nothing was working, it was because I was already just so toxic.

People who scoff at natural remedies usually either haven't tried them, or they are in the same 'toxic body' category as I was. I know people who respond so strongly to a cup of valerian tea that it will knock them out for 12 hours at a stretch. Or they can sniff a little bit of peppermint oil and BOOM, that oncoming migraine is just gone like it never existed. But this never worked for me.

I do not devalue any of these methods at all. I am a firm believer in all of them, actually. I have dozens of friends who have had great luck with Reiki and acupuncture, aromatherapy, and even sound healing. But my body just didn't cooperate. And if you have tried all these things, and are wondering why nothing has worked yet, it is very likely this is the reason.

So what did I do about it?

I learned how to detoxify. And this was a very long and drawn-out process of learning exactly how to do this properly. Luckily for you, all my twists, turns, and mistakes have helped me build a system that is completely safe and *does* work.

And the best part is, you don't have to spend thousands of dollars at some fancy European company's website to reap all the benefits. A lot of the stuff will already be in your house, or as close as the nearest grocery store. Of course, for those of you who do want to go a little deeper with it, there may be some online orders required, but nothing too pricey.

These cleanses are just as effective as the expensive ones. But we don't need a bunch of fancy stuff because the less we have to process, the better our bodies will function.

Let's talk about this process more.

DETOXIFICATION

When you make new, healthy lifestyle choices your body and mind are not used to, the detoxification process is inevitable. And sometimes, it can be very unpleasant.

Let me put it this way; you have spent your entire life treating your body a certain way. Most likely filling it with things that were probably not conducive to whole health.

You have probably even put things in and on your body that have hurt it over the years. All that stuff will leave behind residue whether it is physical, emotional, or both.

Some of that stuff might still literally be in or on your body. The effects it had on your body were probably not pleasant over the long run. Even if you didn't notice it at the time—the lasting effects do build up over extended periods.

Now, in order to detox, you have to go through the process of ridding these things from your body. So it has to go through the whole process again, but in *reverse*.

Luckily, the detoxification process is quicker and more effective than the process you went through to toxify yourself. But that also means the detoxification process is significantly more intense. Therefore, the detoxifying can be very tiring and sometimes even sickening.

For these reasons, I never suggest any drastic treatments unless you are very physically and mentally prepared for the side effects.

When I was in my early twenties, I did long juice fasts all the time. I would definitely be tired during the fast itself, but I would always come out of them feeling energized and amazing.

But as the years passed, the fasting got more difficult for me. As the cleanses weakened my physical body, all my existing health issues would become more pronounced. It took me a while to set aside my ego long enough to accept that intense fasting was no longer acceptable for me.

Instead, I came across a detoxifying diet that didn't strip me of my strength or mental capacities.

The diet consisted almost entirely of cultured

vegetables and a little bit of quinoa, amaranth, or millet. I was able to do this cleanse for weeks at a time without getting too weak. There is something for everyone. No matter how much willpower you do or *don't* have!

The detoxification process is going to happen whether you slowly ease yourself in, or dive in all at once. The more intense the cleanse, the more intense the side effects will be. So just keep that in mind.

Because of all the trial and error and chaos I went through trying to figure out the cleansing process for myself, I now lay out the entire process in a step-by-step format for you here. This has been a long process over the years of discovering which organs need to be cleaned in which order. Also, gentle cleanses are absolutely necessary to keep this process wholly safe and effective.

I must also point out the students in my program go through extensive testing and consultations before the cleansing process. It is absolutely essential that you seek help from a specialist and don't do any drastic cleansing without supervision.

As I said, I used to do long and drastic fasts all the time when I was younger, but eventually, my body couldn't handle it anymore. It turned out I was just stressing my system. So once again, referring to the car metaphor; you have to start from the inside and work your way out.

Many people try doing liver cleanses but don't understand that their livers can't filter everything properly if the other organs aren't working, because then there is no place for the bile to go. The same is true if your colon is completely clogged. There is a specific step-by-step process the organs need to go through so that everything can cleanse in the proper order. If you think about it, it is best to start from the bottom and work your way up.

Your intestines are the final filtration process that your digestive tract sends your food through. Many things can go wrong with the organs, but it usually starts deep inside, and the colon is usually (not always, but usually) the last thing to malfunction. Therefore, you know if your colon is having problems, that means all your other organs are as well. Because by the time it gets to your colon. Everything has already gotten really out of whack.

So imagine you get your liver nice and clean. But where is all that dirty nastiness going to go after it gets pushed out? If your colon is clogged and the nerve endings are sluggish and not working, your colon can't push the rest of that toxic stuff out. So all that ickiness you just cleaned out of your liver is now just stuck at the top of your colon. Just sitting there. Being toxic.

Another unfortunate example of this would be a parasite cleanse. All of us are carrying parasites of some kind. And some are a lot worse than others. For me, I have had a lot of issues with parasites because of my world travels. I have definitely picked up some interesting things—other than gifts for my friends and family! My first instinct is always to come back to my home and do a parasite cleanse.

So I killed off all of these entities in my body, and then I just had dead parasites in my system. But the filtration system in my body wasn't able to handle all these dead parasites, so these disgusting, rotting parasite carcasses were just sitting in my system—unable to go anywhere. And then they would just putrefy.

Lovely, right?

While it is true a dead parasite is not feeding off you directly like a live one, it is still just as bad to have in your body. Therefore, a parasite cleanse isn't necessarily a great idea until you know it will make it through your body's entire filtration system.

Clean the fuel filter!

This is why I strongly suggest you start with preparing the entire digestive tract by softening everything up. Once everything in the gastrointestinal tract has been stirred up and softened and ready to move out, I start with the colon and work my way up. This is my process...

DIGESTIVE TRACT RECONDITIONING

Now, keep in mind, the digestive process actually begins the moment you *smell* food. This will cause your mouth to start watering, and that saliva is part of the digestion process; it is full of enzymes that begin to break the food down. Now, from the moment the food touches the tip of your tongue, everything kicks into gear and doesn't end until it hits the toilet bowl.

You chew it up, it travels down your esophagus when you swallow, and then works its way into the stomach. Remember, the stomach has no teeth, so you need to make sure you chewed that food *really well!*

Your saliva has started the breakdown process in the mouth, so by the time it gets to your stomach, the digestive process should already have begun to take place. The stomach's job is to swish it around using stomach acid to break the food down even further. Therefore, people who deal with things like ulcers are usually suffering from an *lack* of stomach acid, rather than an overabundance (like many believe). Having a good quantity of stomach acid is actually a good thing because that means it can digest your food efficiently.

The first step I highly recommend in digestive reconditioning is *oil pulling*. Perhaps you have heard of it, but you may only know about its positive effects in dental hygiene.

Many people who practice oil pulling don't even realize how important it is for their digestive systems. The reason this triggers the digestive tract is that you are putting a healthy fat in your mouth and swishing it around. You want to do this for at least 10 minutes without swallowing it, and then spit it out. I use sesame oil (just make sure it's not toasted sesame oil, and it's organic). Many people still use coconut oil, but I prefer sesame oil because of its tremendous positive effects on healing the gum lining in the mouth.

Not only does oil pulling kill bacteria in the mouth and help repair the tissues and the membranes, but it triggers your body's digestive tract to start producing digestive enzymes, get saliva flowing, and basically, wake up your digestive system to know that it's time to start processing.

I do an oil pull every single morning right after my first cup of hot water before anything else goes in my mouth. On the rare occasion I miss a day, I can feel it immediately in my body with how I digest my food. I feel bloated and sluggish after eating breakfast. So oil pulling can honestly do wonders, and I highly recommend you try it out.

Now for the filtration system; this is the part that comes after the stomach has started to break everything down. Things begin to filter through your gallbladder, liver, kidneys, and of course, your intestines. The liver's job is to produce bile, so the liver/gallbladder relationship is particularly synergistic.

LIVER/GALLBLADDER

Let's talk about the gallbladder. How many of us really even know what it is or what it does? Or how dramatically important it is for the body's overall health?

Cleansing the liver of gallstones will dramatically

improve digestion. And because digestion is the root of the body's whole health, this is vitally important.

An improperly functioning digestive system can lead to allergies and an inability for the skin to stay hydrated. So by cleansing the gallbladder, we can expect an improvement in these symptoms and our skin to look hydrated and rejuvenated. No more dryness or itching!

Also, when we suffer from shoulder, upper arm, and upper back pain, this can also be linked to a malfunctioning gallbladder. So cleansing the gallbladder can not only reduce pain but also lead to more energy and an increased sense of well-being.

The liver's job is to make bile. At least one to one and a half quarts every day! This interesting little organ is full of tubes which are known as biliary tubing. These tubes deliver the bile to one large tube, which is the common bile duct. The gallbladder is attached to the common bile duct and serves as a storage facility for the incoming bile.

When we eat fats and proteins, this triggers the gallbladder to squeeze itself empty after about 20 minutes. Then the stored bile travels down the common bile duct into the intestines. But for many of us, and this even includes children, the biliary tubing is clogged with gallstones.

Many of us have no symptoms at all from this. But some people develop allergies or hives or more severe problems like an inability to stay hydrated, brain fog, dizziness, headaches, and much more. The problem is that even if we go to a doctor to get scanned or x-rayed, nothing is even visible. This is because the stones are not actually in the gallbladder, or they're just so small they may not have calcified yet. And, in order to be seen in an x-ray, there must be a large amount of calcification.

There are many varieties of gallstones, and most of them have cholesterol crystals in them. These stones can be black, red, white, green, or tan. The green ones are coated with bile.

When the stones grow and multiply, they can cause pressure on the liver, and this will, in turn, cause it to produce less bile. This can also slow the flow of lymphatic fluid. Imagine filling a bottle of water with marbles and then trying to drink it. Less water is able to flow, so it would be difficult to squirt the water into your mouth. This is the case with gallstones.

When gallstones are present, less cholesterol is able to leave the body. This can cause an obvious rise in cholesterol levels. Because gallstones are porous, they can pick up bacteria, cysts, viruses, and parasites that are traveling through the liver.

This can lead to infection forming in a mass which will then continuously supply the body with fresh bacteria and parasites. For people who suffer from stomach infections such as ulcers or intestinal bloating or parasites, they can never find a permanent cure until they relieve the gallstones from the liver.

So many people who are dealing with chronic pain, and suffering from diseases from which they think there is no cure, have no idea that much of their problem lies in these tiny little gallstones.

But the good news is, that cleansing your liver of gallstones is not only easy but completely painless. As well as safe and very effective.

INGREDIENTS YOU WILL NEED ARE:

- Epsom salts
- Olive oil
- Fresh pink grapefruit (or other sour fruit)
- Apple Juice
- A pint jar with a lid for the oil mixture
- A quart jar for the Epsom salt mixture
- One large plastic straw (optional)

Choose a convenient day to do this cleanse. For instance, if you work weekdays, begin the cleanse on a Friday or Saturday so that you'll be able to rest the following day.

If you can avoid it, take no medicines, vitamins, or pills.

Eat a completely fat-free breakfast and lunch, such as oatmeal, fruit, vegetables, salad—anything with no fat. This will allow the bile to build up and apply pressure in the liver. The more pressure that builds up, the more stones will be pushed through the tubing.

If you are able to fast the whole day, please do so. You may still drink apple juice throughout the day.

Around 2 p.m.:

Eat a light meal and drink only water and apple juice for the rest of the night. If you are hypoglycemic, small amounts of lean meat are okay. Otherwise, avoid fat completely. Fruits and vegetables are recommended.

Prepare your full Epsom salt mixture. This will make four doses.

Mix three cups of water or apple juice with two tablespoons of Epsom salts.

Shake and put in the refrigerator.

6 p.m.:

Drink one serving. This is only one-quarter of the cold Epsom salt mixture that you prepared earlier. It tastes TERRIBLE, so use the plastic straw if you need to to help you get it down (I just plug my nose).

8 p.m.:

Drink another serving.

. . .

10:15 P.M.:

Be sure that you have completed everything you need to do before bed already. This next step should take place immediately before getting in bed.

Pour a half-cup of olive oil into the pint jar.

Wash the grapefruit and squeeze three-quarters of a cup of the juice into a jar. The pulp is okay, too.

Close the jar tightly and shake until it gets watery. The grapefruit will emulsify the oil.

*If you are allergic to grapefruit you can use lemon, pineapple, or sour apple instead.

Be sure to go to the bathroom before you drink your mixture because you will go to bed immediately after you drink it.

Drink the mixture while standing up. Be sure to drink the entire thing within two minutes.

Lay down immediately, because the sooner you do, the more stones you will be able to release.

Lie flat on your back, or on your right side, with your head propped up on some pillows. Remain perfectly still for at least 20 minutes.

Here it helps to visualize the process of this cleansing medicine traveling through your digestive tract and removing the stones. You may even be able to feel the stones traveling along the bile duct.

There is no pain because the Epsom salt mixture opened the bile ducts. After 20 minutes, relax and go to sleep.

. . .

QAT WANDERS

The following morning, after 6 a.m., take your third dose of Epsom salts immediately upon waking. But wait until you feel okay (if you had any indigestion or nausea—which ranges from mild to severe depending on the person). At this point, you may go back to bed. Drink as much water as you like now.

After this dose, wait two hours and then take a half-cup of the oil mixture. Lay back down for 30 minutes or more if you like.

Allow another two hours to pass before you take another dose of the Epsom salts. This will increase the number of stones you remove. If you feel like you've had more than enough, that is fine. Go ahead and give it a rest.

After another two more hours have passed, go ahead and eat. Start with apple juice. Then maybe a little bit of fruit 30 minutes later. An hour after the fruit, eat a light meal. By the afternoon, you should feel more rejuvenated. (In some cases, the discomfort will last another day or so; it depends on how clogged your system was to begin with.)

Expect diarrhea first thing in the morning. As well as a number of loose bowel movements throughout the day. If you are really brave, you can look in the toilet and swish off the top layer of sludge with some toilet paper to see the gallstones sitting in the bottom of the toilet.

If you examine them, notice what color and size they are. If the bile duct was clogged with cholesterol crystals that did not form into round stones, they will appear like a puffy foam floating on top of the toilet water. This is just as important to purge.

THIS PROCESS MAY NEED TO BE REPEATED OCCASIONALLY to completely flush the digestive tract. Depending on how much toxicity we may have accumulated or how sick we are when we start.

It is possible that while the first cleanse may rid the body of many stones, sometimes they are not all removed, and sometimes they only travel further through the tubes, so some of the same symptoms may come back again in a few days (in which case, the process needs to be repeated).

Keep in mind that everybody is different. Feel free to repeat the cleanse every month until a full recovery takes place. But absolutely do *not* practice this cleanse while suffering from acute liver pain!

This is a very safe cleanse that has been conducted safely even on elderly individuals. No one has reported pain, but some have reported feeling slightly different for a day or two afterward. Most people claim to feel lighter, cleaner, and more energized.

While gallstones are thought to be formed in the gallbladder instead of the liver, this is actually not the case. It is also not widely known that there are actually hundreds of tiny, soft stones, rather than just a few hard ones, as many claim.

While gallstones are not connected to any kind of pain, they can cause an obstruction, which can shock the body into feeling pain.

This is why the softer stones are unknown because, by the time acute gallstone pain attacks happen, the gallstones have already made their way to the gallbladder and are now large and calcified enough to be seen on an x-ray.

At this point, unfortunately, people tend to visit the emergency room which leads to surgical removal from the gallbladder. This takes care of the large stones, but the obstructions and digestive problems will remain because the softer stones were not handled.

This is why cleansing the gallbladder regularly is so crucial to the overall health of the body.

Once your liver and gallbladder are nice and happy, you are ready to move on to the colon.

COLON

So here's a fun question. What does your poop say about you?

The answer: quite a bit! Or at least about your health anyway. But remember, physical, mental, and spiritual health are all interrelated. They feed off of each other, relate to each other, and are affected by one another.

So let's get back to poop.

A healthy colon means a healthy digestive tract, which means a healthy body, which means a healthy mind, which means a healthy spirit.

So I can guarantee that if you are dealing with chronic pain, you need to clean your colon. However, first, we need to figure out what your colon actually needs. The way to do that is to take a good look at your poop.

Yes, that's right.

You also need to pay attention to your pooping schedule. Are you regular? Do you even know what regular is? I have worked with clients who actually thought one bowel movement per week was normal! Not kidding.

Ideally, you should be going one to three times per day! It should be well-formed, a medium-brown color, and you should have a clean wipe, meaning it shouldn't take you 10 minutes to wipe yourself clean. It should also come out of your body within seconds of sitting on the toilet. If you have to sit there for a while, or if you're grunting and breathing hard, then you're constipated.

If it is divided into little sections or pellets that come out one at a time, then you are constipated! Or, if it is black or you see whole, undigested food—guess what—constipated!

Constipation means your body is dehydrated. And dehydration is super dangerous for your entire inner system. Hot water is such an essential first step because many people are getting plenty of fluids, but their bodies are still dehydrated because their colons aren't absorbing it properly.

I know this because it happened to me. My colon wasn't able to absorb any of the nutrients or the liquid I was putting into it. So even though I was drinking more than a gallon of fluid per day, I was dehydrated all the time. You could see it in my skin, my hair, my eyes, and yes . . . my poop.

On the other hand, if you have frequent diarrhea or soft, squishy bowel movements, this doesn't necessarily mean you're hydrated either. First of all, if you are literally pooping out liquid, then you are apparently not hydrated because that's where all your fluid is going. If a bowel movement is an overly messy process for you (you know, like soft-serve ice cream—such a lovely thought), then your body is overly acidic. Once again, this doesn't mean you have too much stomach acid as most people think, it just means you are too acidic.

KIDNEYS

Once we have completed the previous cleansing steps, it is time to flush the kidneys and bladder. This is one of the easiest things to do, but there is also some preventive maintenance that should take place after the flush.

The easiest thing you can do first is—you guessed it—hot water. Your best bet is actually just to give up food altogether for at least 24 hours and drink nothing but hot water, but if you're hypoglycemic, and this just isn't an option for you, then, by all means, don't fast. Just overload your system with water.

If you're used to taking supplements, don't even bother. They're just going to get flushed out because you're going to be drinking so much water everything is going to go out with it. Cranberry juice is also always a good option and very well known. Just make sure it's not made from concentrate or mixed with other juices that are usually full of sugar.

When I do a cranberry juice flush, I mix it with water and also a little bit of liquid stevia to sweeten it. Stevia is an excellent option for repairing the digestive tract because it is a fantastic sweetening alternative with no sugar in it. Therefore, there is nothing for the yeast to feed off of, and it won't aggravate inflammation.

There is also a drink I like to make when I'm doing a kidney flush that involves apple cider or coconut vinegar, lemon or lime juice, stevia, Celtic salt, and water. I drink about two to three quarts of that mixture over the course of a day for three days. It is very nourishing for the kidneys, and it will help clean the bladder safely. Do be warned, though, if you have a sensitive tummy it can cause nausea.

But as for the preventive maintenance, know that caffeine is the biggest contender to kidney problems next to sugar and artificial, processed ingredients. Caffeine affects your liver, gallbladder, colon, and heart as well, but I put it here with the kidneys because they are usually the first things to have noticeable problems related to caffeine. Alcohol will do the same thing. So just keep that in mind.

If you drink 10 cups of coffee in the morning and no liquid (this is why I always start with hot water to begin to nourish and hydrate the digestive tract), you are making your kidneys work harder than they are capable of working. So if you can—give up caffeine for a little while, just until you get your kidneys clean and working efficiently.

A helpful way to limit the negative effects of the caffeine would be for every cup of coffee (or whatever caffeinated beverage you drink) make sure you drink a cup of hot water before and after. This will help offset the detrimental effects it can have on your kidneys.

HEAVY METALS

Last but not least, it is crucial to strip out some of the toxic effects from unavoidable exposure to heavy metals. Many people don't realize just how much heavy metal content is inside their bodies and just how much harm it is doing. Even though it is unavoidable, it is possible to minimize the effects. It is also relatively easy and manageable when done over an extended period.

I personally recommend is zeolite. It only takes a tablespoon per day and it is fantastic at clearing out the system. Many of the parasites that have taken up residence in the body also thrive with the heavy metals, so the zeolite is helpful for this, too.

Diatomaceous earth and bentonite clay are also effective, as is activated charcoal. None of these things are costly, and even though they are not necessarily tasty, they don't have much of a flavor (but they do have a weird chalk-like consistency). A couple of tablespoons a day for a few weeks is all that is necessary, and this can be done three to four times per year. Some people like to take it every day, that is up to you, but I do not personally like to do things daily because the body can become desensitized to it. But it is a great option for cleaning out your system painlessly.

However, if you do take too much, it can also cause nausea and diarrhea. So start with a little bit and work your way up. I recommend doing this after the rest of the organs have been cleansed, because this will sweep up living and dead parasites, as well as heavy metals, and it will absorb and pull out leftover toxins in the entire digestive tract as it goes through. So it is more efficient when done after everything else has been cleaned out because it's kind of like the final sweep through the system to get all those last little bits out.

Do not, however, take this within 30 minutes of eating anything that would be considered high in nutrients or minerals. Because these particular things do draw *everything* out of the system. These drawing powders pull *everything* out of the digestive tract and shoot it through. So if you are to take any kind of herb or mineral supplement along with it, your body will have no way to absorb it.

MICROBIOME

The microbiome is the inner ecosystem that lives in our digestive tracts. According to Yoga, in conjunction with Ayurveda, there are some basic guidelines for food to increase in your diet. There are also foods to reduce or avoid. Just remember that everyone's body is different, and what is medicine for one could be poison to another. That is obviously quite an extreme, but just keep your own personal needs in mind as you look over this list.

Increase:

- Fresh, whole fruits.
- All vegetables, except for an abundant amount of onions or garlic.
- Mung beans or lentils.
- Nuts and seeds like almonds, coconut, or sesame. Preferably raw and soaked.
- Plant-based oils like sesame, coconut, or ghee.

Raw and unrefined.
- Organic or raw dairy products from cows or goats. Especially warm milk with turmeric and nutmeg, yogurt, and cottage cheese (limit hard cheeses).
- Organic whole grains with minimal processing.
- Herbal teas and spring water.
- Sweet spices such as cardamom, fennel, cinnamon, turmeric, or mint.

Reduce:

- Meat.
- Canned food.
- Garlic and onions.
- Extremely spicy food.
- Fried food.

Avoid:

- Commercial dairy.
- Refined sugar and flour.
- Artificial sweeteners.
- Aspartame.
- Tap water.
- Genetically engineered food.
- Artificially flavored or processed food.

Now, don't let this list overwhelm you. If you drink wine sometimes or still eat meat, it certainly doesn't make you a bad or unhealthy person.

Also, know there is a lot of science behind this for each individual. And not everything on this list is good for everyone. Especially those who are just embarking on the healing process. This is why I feel a personalized action plan is absolutely crucial for someone preparing a sequence of cleansing.

This is just a framework that Yoga and Ayurveda have given us that I wanted to share with you. I personally do not follow all these guidelines strictly either, although I tried for years. In all honesty, if my body was not so sensitive, I may not even follow all the guidelines I do now.

Fasting is less effective if we cannot completely remove the desire for food. So just remember, there is no need to shock the body. Be kind to it and conscious of it, and in return, it will be kind to you.

THE CLEAN SWEEP

Now here is the entire process in a short sequential break down:

- Begin to prime the digestive tract by reconditioning it. Soften everything up by balancing the microbiome to try to recover homeostasis. Start with daily oil pulling and lots of hot water.

- Nourish the colon, but remember, things are not going to make their way to the colon from the top down if you have a malfunctioning system. You have to start from the bottom and work your way up. Try warm-water enemas or colon hydrotherapy.
- Once your colon is functioning correctly, you can cleanse the liver and gallbladder. Now, remember that gallstones are actually created in the liver, and many times you can't even tell they are there and they won't show up on an x-ray. But almost everyone is carrying them. Soften these up and get them ready to move.
- Once energy levels start to improve, you can be reasonably certain the liver is happy. Then you can move to the kidneys. Once again, remember cold water goes straight to your bladder, so nourish the kidneys with warm to hot water. This is the point where you want to flush everything out with watered down cranberry juice and/or the vinegar drink I mentioned earlier.
- Now that you have given specific attention to each organ, it is time to nourish the colon from the top down. This, in turn, sustains the rest of the digestive tract. But start with

> things specific for the colon. Use the parasite-drawing powders and senna tea (use caution with the tea and be sure to follow the instructions on the package).

There may be a lot of gas and bloating throughout this, as well as diarrhea, but constipation shouldn't be an issue. Once you have cleared out constipation, you should be feeling better.

But what is going to keep everything from happening all over again?

The answer is...

THE ANTI-YEAST/ANTI-INFLAMMATION DIET

In order to keep this happy microbiome going, now it's time for general maintenance. We need to starve the yeast in the body and lower the inflammation.

I promise this is easier than it sounds. I did this successfully in a matter of weeks, and I know hundreds of others who have as well. Now, depending on how much candida and inflammation you have in your body (which I personally had quite a lot), it could take less time, or it could take more time.

Keep in mind, I had pretty chronic candidiasis, and I was still able to get the condition relatively under control in a matter of weeks. And after several months, I was able to eradicate the problem altogether. This does require some willpower and discipline at the beginning, however, because the only way to starve the yeast is to cut out anything the yeast can feed off of from your diet. Mostly sugar or anything that breaks down into sugar, such as carbs and starches.

Random fact about me: I was on a vegan diet for a rather long time, and I was doing it specifically for health and compassion reasons. I want to live a life as free from cruelty as physically possible. Hence the appeal of a diet void of animal products. Now keep in mind, I am a researcher. I read everything I can get my hands on if I'm doing something because I want to make sure I'm doing it for the right reasons, and I don't screw it up. If I do, I learned from my mistakes. So hopefully this will spare you some trouble now because this is what happened:

I was careful to make sure I was getting all my proper nutrient levels. I was getting plenty of protein, by the way. Just in case you're one of those people who think that is such a huge deal, especially with vegan diets. I don't need to hear, "You probably weren't getting enough protein!" *Seriously, so tired of that.*

I did my best to stay hydrated, and I was physically active. For the first portion of being vegan, I had plenty of energy—that was never an issue. I couldn't imagine why anyone *wouldn't* be vegan because I felt so amazing!

Except for the gas and bloating. For the longest time I thought it was just my body detoxing. Because everything I was hearing and reading told me that digestive issues like that take place when you are going through a detoxification process.

After all those years of eating junk food as a child, my body was just trying to get clean. But this went on for years. *Way too many years.*

How long was I supposed to be detoxing? And eventually, the gas and bloating turned into straight-up pain. I talked about this earlier, so I won't recap all the digestive problems. But they weren't pretty, to say the least. I had more than one doctor tell me I needed to start eating meat again. I brushed this off because I didn't want to eat a dead animal. That was just disgusting.

But as the paleo and the ketogenic diets started to rise in popularity, I started doing some more research. I wanted to understand why people were so adamant about this. To this day, I don't abide by any particular diet. Honestly, I still find most of these diets to be passing fads. Even the vegan diet to an extent. Keep in mind, I was mostly doing the *raw* vegan thing for a while, but this made me feel so sick it was ridiculous.

I later discovered that someone with my constitution isn't necessarily meant to eat raw foods all the time unless they're doing a cleanse. So once I started eating more cooked food, I started getting better. This was so weird to me because it was the opposite of everything I knew.

Raw foods are alive! They're supposed to be the healthiest! And there is still a lot of truth behind this. The issue for me was that my body was already so toxic, it couldn't digest these healthy foods I was eating. Yes, raw foods are very healthy, but the problem is they're also very difficult to digest, especially if your digestive tract has absolutely no idea what it's doing!

Now the same is true with almost all foods that fall into the vegan category. Beans, nuts, and grains are all tough for a low-functioning microbiome to process. Your body just freaks out when you stick the stuff in there and overcompensates with gas. Have you ever heard of a constipated vegan? Well, now you have.

I won't go into all the ridiculous things I tried to keep my moral values with my diet, so to cut a long story short, I discovered the magic of a gut-healing diet. The most prominent issue for me at the time was that all the gut-healing diets I could find involved meat or at least some sort of animal product.

So after much inner turmoil, I started eating fish. Eventually, I also added bone broth and collagen into my diet. I realize that this may ruffle some feathers now. I'm sure that some of you reading this right now are avid vegetarians or vegans. I get it. I was too.

But something that helped me was reading a book written by His Holiness the Dalai Lama. In his memoir, *Freedom in Exile*, he talked about some severe health issues he was having. He went to many traditional Eastern doctors, and they were all telling him his body wasn't equipped to be vegetarian. This pained and saddened him because he didn't want to start eating meat. His true religion is compassion, after all. But after becoming deathly ill, and having enough prompting from his followers that his life is more important, he agreed to start taking portions of meat.

He still offered thanks when he ate it, and he wouldn't eat anything that would be killed specifically for him. But he also recognized the fact that he, as a human—especially as the Dalai Lama—was going to be able to do a lot more for the universal vibration than the animals that were feeding him.

This, in turn, also assists in the animals themselves accumulating good karma because they were dying for a purpose and feeding the Dalai Lama; therefore also assisting in raising the vibration of the world on a global level.

Now I am not in any way saying that if you are a vegetarian you should go out there and start eating meat now. I am still a firm believer that a vegetarian lifestyle is ideal in many aspects. So if you are a vegetarian or vegan, I would like to personally thank you for the positive impact you have on our world!

However, for me, right now, in this stage in my life, I have had to set aside my ego. I have accepted that my ego was a big part of my wanting to stay vegetarian. I have had to do what I have come to understand is necessary to keep my body functioning at optimal levels.

I can't serve humanity very well if I can barely get out of bed!

I do not partake in animal products very often, and I

avoid them as much as I can. When I do take animal products now, I try to make sure they're as ethically sourced as possible. I also give thanks to not only the universe and Divine Source, but to the animal itself (and the animal's soul) that gave its physical life to help me become healthier.

I do still believe that eating animals—especially creatures that suffered to death or were tortured—does indeed lower your vibration. From the inside out. This is why I think it is so important to find ethically sourced animal products. But I also believe that giving thanks and blessing your food (I also like to chant my mantra while I eat) raises the vibration of that food as well. And when we take things into our body with gratitude and a preconceived belief that only good things will come from it, then it will actually nourish our bodies and benefit us.

I have to admit I struggled with guilt for a very long time because of this. I now do my best to accept what has been placed before me on this earth. If I eat something that I know isn't necessarily ideal for me, I still just give thanks and take it with gratitude. As I consume it, I chant my mantra and continue to give thanks, visualizing it doing only good for my body.

ACTION STEPS

When you eat, tell yourself you are taking only nourishing goodness into your body. Anything that is not conducive to your overall health and well-being is being passed straight through your body and dispelled.

Refer to the recommended diet in the Resources section at the end of this book. Keep in mind, it is important to use discernment when choosing foods that are right for your body. I highly recommend you see a certified Ayurvedic specialist to make sure the recommended foods will be helpful for your body type.

Here are some foods and herbs you can add into your diet to maximize gut health:

- Sauerkraut
- Blueberries
- Kefir
- Coconut oil
- Grass-fed butter
- Bone broth
- Collagen
- Turmeric
- Ginger, cardamom, and fennel (combined)

YOGA WITH SUBCATEGORIES

Perhaps you have been wondering why the book was titled *Overcoming Chronic Pain Through Yoga,* but it has taken me until Chapter 11 to get to the part about Yoga?

The answer:

This entire book has been about Yoga so far. Yoga has a much deeper meaning than many people are aware of. Everything in this book has all consisted of the Yoga of overcoming chronic pain. Yoga translates directly to *union,* or *to yoke.* And because it was never initially intended as just physical exercise, it can be applied to just about any healing modality there is.

This ancient spiritual science has been designed to unite us with our Supreme Self. The Divine Light. Before I go further into healing through Yoga, I want to talk about the eight limbs that comprise the science behind it.

You see, the physical postures are a tiny part. In fact, they aren't even mentioned until the third limb of Yoga. And all of this comprises the science of Yoga, making it essential to know all the limbs before one can even call themselves a Yogi. If the only aspect of Yoga you are familiar with or have tried are the physical postures, which are actually called *asanas*, then you should really just be saying you are practicing Asana. Not Yoga. Yoga is whole and complete. That being said, here is a very short breakdown of the eight limbs.

THE EIGHT LIMBS

The basic ancient principles are just as relevant today as they were thousands of years ago. If applied properly, they can be truly transformative. But to understand these principles at a deeper level will take time and dedication. It also takes an open mind. If you can learn to open your mind, you can learn to open yourself to physical healing as well as open your soul.

This is where we will dive into the eight limbs of Yoga. They are nourished by regular and consistent practice. At this point, we become aware of what we put in our bodies and how we interact with the world around us.

Many people, especially in the West, think of Yoga as physical exercise. But it is so much more than that. Yoga is an ancient science. It was actually broken down into eight limbs many centuries ago. These limbs are:

1. Yama
2. Niyama
3. Asana
4. Pranayama
5. Pratyahara
6. Dharana
7. Dhyana
8. Samadhi

If you want to study the eight limbs further, I suggest you check out the book, *The Tree of Yoga*, by B.K.S. Iyengar.

YAMA: RESTRAINTS

Begins with the control of the organs of one's actions. This is the foundation from which the rest of the limbs can grow.

Yama translates into *ethical disciplines* or non-harming in thought, word, and deed. It all circles around speaking, thinking, and doing kind things.

THE YAMAS INCLUDE:

- Ahimsa - non-violence
- Satya - non-lying
- Asteya - non-stealing
- Brahmacharya - control of sensual pleasure

- Aparigraha - freedom from covetousness

In a nutshell, the Yamas are things one should ideally avoid.

NIYAMA: OBSERVANCES

Control of the organs of perception, or, in other words, these are things we *should* do. Niyama focuses on self-observation, self-discipline, contentment, and self-study.

THE LIST OF NIYAMAS ARE:

- Saucha - cleanliness
- Santosha - contentment
- Tapas - discipline
- Svadhyaya - self-study
- Isvara-pranidhana - self-surrender

ASANA: SEAT OR POSTURE

These are the physical postures. This is frequently the only form of Yoga people are aware of, when, in reality, it is only a very small portion of the Yoga practice.

The asanas were designed to maintain the health of the cells in the physical body. When the body becomes healthy, the mind is brought closer to the soul. It is said that one should perform these asanas in such a way as to lead the mind from attachment to the body toward the light of the soul.

PRANAYAMA: BREATHWORK

This is where the respiratory and circulatory systems are brought into a harmonious state.

Pranayama means *breath-control*. We can only extend our bodies to their fullest when we are able to synchronize our movements with our breath cycles. It is important to always remember to breathe deeply when we feel stressed, pain, or when we physically exert ourselves.

Practicing breathwork is purifying and invigorating. The more we practice, the deeper we are able to breathe. The average person is a very shallow breather, using only a small percentage of his or her actual lung capacity. By bringing attention to this, we eventually allow ourselves to open up more. On average, a Yoga practitioner who has been practicing for more than a year can bring in a quart of air more than the average person. We want to learn to breathe deeper and deeper with time.

PRATYAHARA: INTROSPECTION

Withdrawal of the senses. The inward journey of the senses from the outer body to the inner being. The core.

The attunement with the soul. While simultaneously beginning to filter out all outside distractions.

Pratyahara is focusing on being present and having a single-minded focus. This is an act of going against the current of desire and memory in the mind. Desires and memories like to swoop into our consciousness and try to take over.

Desires force us to dwell in the future, where memories force us to dwell in the past. If we can deny these forces of nature, then we can remain in the present.

We can go deep within ourselves. With the help of introspection, we can observe our thoughts and actions from an outsider's perspective. These observances give us the intelligence to act on a level of the soul and detach from the affairs of the world. We must learn to cleanse the consciousness and free it from the possessive clutches of our thoughts.

DHARANA: CONCENTRATION

Focusing the attention on the core of the being. A strong journey inward that allows a single-pointed focus on the inner self, void of distractions. Through our practice of sense withdrawal, we develop better concentration, not only on our mats but in all aspects of life as well. It is complete and single-pointed attention. Deliberate attention. Being fully aware. And this awareness leads directly into the next step.

DHYANA: MEDITATION

This is when the observer and the observed are united as one. It is the experience of unity. An attainment that is void of thought or perception.

It is contemplation. Full awareness through your whole being. It is not emptiness as many think. It is fullness. When we sleep, we are empty. So if meditation were emptiness, we would all be much more evolved after sleeping for eight hours every night!

Meditation does not mean just emptying your mind. You can empty yourself of all thoughts, while still remaining fully aware. This is a dynamic balance between the inner and outer consciousness.

You may have some experience with meditation, but it takes hours and hours of practice regularly over many years to reach a true meditative state into which you can reach the final limb.

SAMADHI: UNITY

A state of joy and peace. It is thought to only come after study, practice, and focus on each of the other limbs. They were designed to help you refine and develop all these important pieces so that you can essentially reach extraordinary peace and happiness.

One cannot achieve this state until all the previous steps have been mastered. This is when the soul is finally integrated into each and every part of the body.

This is where the body, the mind, and the soul are all united as one and merge with the divine presence; the universal spirit.

AND THERE YOU HAVE IT. AN EXCEEDINGLY BRIEF explanation of the eight limbs of Yoga. I highly recommend looking further into this subject because it is truly fascinating. Having such an ethereal concept broken down into such a step-by-step, scientific process was very helpful for me in coming to understand the essence of Yoga in my young, overly analytical mind. These principles go hand in hand with the concepts of Ayurveda, which is just as old.

THE PRACTICE

If you have ever attended a "Yoga class" you are familiar with the physical postures. And some of you might also be familiar with some of the spirituality behind it as well. It is becoming exceedingly popular in Yoga classes, even in the West nowadays, to include bits and pieces of the other limbs of Yoga into the sequences.

It is no longer uncommon to come across practices in Yoga classes such as the use of mudras, mantra, and Pranayama. If these things sound strange to you; don't worry, I'm going to explain a little, but there is also a multitude of resources out there about these different subjects and how they directly correlate to certain types of pain.

MUDRAS ESPECIALLY, CAN BE VERY BENEFICIAL. THERE IS a tremendous amount of nerve endings in the fingertips. The human nervous system is an amazingly complex network. There are some specific parts of the body where the nerve endings give off a particularly concentrated amount of energy.

The fingertips are the most-known example, but also, the tips of the toes and the tip of the tongue. Not only do you give off energy from these areas, but you receive it as well. This is a reason that "French kissing" is so intimate. By touching the tip of your tongue to someone else's, you are experiencing an energy exchange that can be even more intimate than sex. This is why you feel comfortable kissing your significant other that way, but not a relative!

The tips of the fingers and the toes are other examples, but because the toes are not quite as bendable, the fingers are used significantly more often for mudras (which is energetically aligned fingertip placement). You can touch fingertips with another person and feel an intense energy transfer, but you can also do this when you are by yourself.

When you place your hands and fingers into specific positions, you can line up the meridians of your body in a very purposeful fashion. And this can have straightforward and intentional results.

You can also direct your focus toward specific areas of the body, for instance, there is a mudra explicitly designed for the health of the pelvis. Also, the joining of the palms epitomizes the right and left hemispheres of the brain, representing unification. The many nerves endings in the palms make them very sensitive. By placing them together in Namaste Mudra (or prayer position), you can change your chemistry to foster love within. This unity is the origin of life. Integration of this energy can facilitate us to give our best to society through love.

There is a fabulous book I came across many years ago called *Mudras: Yoga in Your Hands,* by Gertrud Hirschi, I highly recommend to anyone interested and learning more about this.

MANTRA IS ANOTHER PRACTICE THAT HAS BECOME A BIG part of my life. We talked about affirmations, and this is just a more intricate version. A mantra has been specially designed (many of them are thousands of years old) in the ancient Sanskrit language to hold certain vibrational frequencies to achieve a desired result. Sometimes the desired effect is world peace, or health of the body, or union with God.

There are mantras designed to channel specific Hindu deities in the Hindu religion, such as Ganesha, who is the remover of obstacles, or Vishnu, the preserver. When repeated over and over, 108 times (which is the number of beads on a *mala*), the mantra builds more power. This type of power is emitted out into the universe once again, raising the vibration.

Another variation of this would be in the Catholic church with a rosary and Hail Mary. This idea is in no way unique. People have been utilizing the magnificent power of words since the beginning of time. Another quick note about mantra is that each chakra has a corresponding seed-syllable mantra. Which basically just means one syllable. If you are interested in knowing more about chakras, I talk about them more in my previous book, *Yoga for YOU*.

When you repeatedly chant the seed-syllable for the corresponding chakra, you activate and balance that chakra. Therefore, if you recite all seven syllables in order, you build energy from the base chakra all the way up to the crown over and over again. This creates an energetic vibrational loop throughout your body.

Chanting the sacred syllable, *Om*, is another example of this. Creating these vibrations has tremendous healing ability and will leave you feeling better and better the more you do it. Mainly because, the more you become attuned to these things, the more sensitive your body becomes to these types of healing energies.

Remember how I said that a toxic body doesn't respond well to alternative healing modalities? Even though I believe so firmly in Reiki, I didn't feel a thing when I went to my sessions because my body was too toxic, and my energy was too closed off.

But the cleaner my body gets, the better I feel, and the more sensitive I become to energy and higher vibrational frequencies. I can actually *feel* my vibration getting higher as I move forward through life. I genuinely wish to help others raise their vibrations as well, because if we can all raise our vibrations, the higher the global vibration will be! And Earth becomes a better place. If that's not motivation, then I don't know what it is.

SEQUENCING

Coming back to the Yoga postures now; sequencing is incredibly important. The asanas are meant to be practiced in particular orders to achieve optimal energetic flow. And since each pose activates different parts of the body, it is essential to understand the body's roadmap well enough to direct energy to the right places in the proper order.

A really good and well-educated Yoga instructor knows these factors and applies them to every class they teach. Unfortunately, I have been to numerous classes taught by poorly educated teachers who knew nothing about sequencing or even proper alignment.

The first thing to note is that every pose has a counterpose. When you do a forward bend, you should follow it with a backbend. When you twist to the right, you should twist to the left. If you do a balancing sequence, you should start with core strengthening. I regularly see classes end with core strengthening or incorporate several backbends in a row, followed by a twist or just the final lying down posture (known as Corpse Pose or *Savasana*)—not okay!

Now I want to talk about stretching the opposite muscles than the ones which are hurting (I will go into more detail about this in the next chapter), this is related to the counterpose system in Yoga. As I said, Yoga (Union) is designed to balance and unite the body, mind, and spirit. It joins male and female aspects, dark and light, hot and cold, dry and moist. All levels of duality.

Yoga is like a cosmic dance. When you push you must pull, what goes up must come down. When you do a sequence of postures that raises energy toward the crown, you must also do a series of positions that reign the energy back down.

When you perform an energizing sequence that gets the heart pumping, you have to follow up with a cooldown after heating it up so much. Balancing these Yin and Yang aspects is crucial for a well-sequenced

Yoga practice. This is why I believe it is so important to study under well-trained Yoga instructors until you learn these concepts intuitively enough to do them yourself.

A few of the Yoga styles I trust (if you are interested in looking into them) would be Iyengar, Jivamukti, and Bikram. These particular forms have been carefully crafted according to the science of the human body and energetic alignment systems. The teachers trained in these particular types have gone through intensive training that is very specific and well-rounded. In order to teach any of these styles of Yoga, they have to be certified by the original creators of that style. This is a gem indeed considering there is no actual requirement at all to teach Yoga in most establishments.

If you want to know more about how to decide on a style of Yoga, check out my first book, *Yoga for YOU*. I go in-depth about the different styles of Yoga and how to choose the best one for you.

Like I said, I had been teaching Yoga for a few years before I ever bothered to get a certification. And even the certification programs nowadays are left wanting. There are studios (which I shall not name) that have created chains across the country and crank out teachers like a gumball machine. These "teachers" are then let loose into the world with no real knowledge of how to keep their students from damaging themselves.

I have been passionate about this subject for a long time. This is why I am so adamant to help my students understand their bodies. Especially if we suffer from chronic pain, many things could go wrong when we attend a typical "Yoga class."

This is why an understanding of not only the fundamentals, but of our personal needs, is essential when attempting any physically demanding activity. But because of the fear (which is just anticipation of future pain) of making the chronic pain worse, many sufferers avoid physical activity altogether. This is actually one of the worst things we can do.

We *need* physical activity. But we need to do it mindfully! It is best to start gently, but then, as we build up momentum, it is very possible—and even encouraged—to push ourselves further and further as our bodies get stronger and healthier. We just need to know our breaking point and avoid coming to it. But with a gentle push, we can overcome chronic pain.

HOT YOGA

This leads me into the topic of hot Yoga, which is wonderful for softening up the muscles, warming up the joints and ligaments, and allowing the body to open and flex more than would be possible in a cooler room.

Depending on the style of the class, the room is typically kept at a temperature anywhere from 90 to 118 degrees Fahrenheit. Hot Yoga opens up your pores and makes you sweat, so that you can detox even faster than you would otherwise, while practicing intense detoxification poses such as twists and inversions.

Some people would consider hot Yoga to be its own style in itself. But I disagree with that. I have taken many different styles of classes in a hot room. I got something different out of each one of them. The only way to determine if hot Yoga is actually a good fit for you (or not) is to try it out at least a few times. But hot Yoga is *not* for everyone, especially those with a tendency toward hypermobility or blood pressure issues. If this is the case in your personal situation, then the next section is for you.

THE BODY IS A TEMPLE SO WHAT WENT WRONG!?

Okay, so let's just be honest. If you are suffering from chronic pain, your body is probably a little screwed up. Maybe a little more than a little. You are hurting. And you don't want to be. It is the essence of human nature to seek pleasure and avoid pain. But when we have been experiencing pain our whole lives, many of us lose interest and the drive to seek pleasure at all. We just want less pain. This goes in line with the feelings of hopelessness. But there really is hope.

Now that you have made it this far in the book, you probably understand that something is misfiring deep down inside you. And maybe if you've already started applying the principles in this book, you have already figured out what it is.

Hopefully, you have started to implement some of the concepts here and are noticing results. If you have started from the inside, things are beginning to improve, and you are starting to feel better. But this doesn't change the fact that something has already gone wrong. We need to minimize the existing damage as much as possible.

DAMAGE CONTROL

Self-awareness usually begins with body awareness. You can have body awareness without self-awareness, but not the other way around. Just start by paying attention to your body. You will notice more and more as you do this. There are some common issues we should start with, though.

I know I said earlier that I'm not a huge fan of telling people what *not* to do. But there are definitely some tendencies and habits we pick up which are not conducive to our overall well-being. In fact, doing these things repeatedly can cause—or already has caused—a lot of damage. But the good news is they can be corrected. So instead of looking at this as being told what *not* to do, try looking at it as an opportunity to make a positive change and try new things to develop further beneficial habits.

There are a few things we can look out for with a teeny bit of self-awareness. There are some things we can avoid doing in our day-to-day activities if we are just mindful enough to think about it. Things like standing with our toes pointing outward or inward or *walking* like that for that matter. This is one of those habits that shoots the pelvis out of alignment. Slouching is an obvious one, but interestingly enough, so is standing up *too straight*. Both of these can cause our breath to become entirely too shallow.

Eating late at night is another big one. Most of us already know this, but how many of us honestly abide by it? This doesn't have a direct effect on our skeletal and muscular alignment, though... Or does it?

The thing is, when it comes to eating late at night, we are filling up our digestive systems and expecting them to work through the night. Even though the rest of the body is trying to rest. Our digestive tracts need time to rest as well. It goes into a sluggish state when we sleep.

Therefore, the foods we eat within five hours before bed remain in our digestive tracts and do not go through thoroughly or efficiently while we sleep. This is why so many of us wake up with heartburn or nausea in the mornings. But what many people don't think about is what this does to the rest of our bodies. That food won't get much further than the small intestine where it tends to get stuck if the body is in a reclining position.

There are so many twists and turns and pockets throughout the entire intestinal tract, it makes it virtually impossible for a sluggish digestive system (which is what it is while you are sleeping) to push the food through completely. This causes the food to back up and get stored in these little pockets and start to putrefy.

We become literally *full of crap*. This causes inflammation and swelling in the area, and eventually, pressure on the pelvis and the nerves, muscles, bones, and tissues around it. This can have a very unpleasant effect on the spinal structure as well as the posture. And it can throw us completely out of alignment if we tend to sleep on one side every night.

Because the food builds up only on that side of the body, it can cause things to get entirely out of whack, throwing your spinal and pelvic alignment to one side or the other. And I didn't even touch on how bloated and uncomfortable this makes us look and feel.

Speaking of how detrimental lying in a prone position can be for your gastrointestinal tract and your overall physical alignment; I would like to bring to light another myth that many people believe when it comes to back pain. So here's the truth: **resting your back for prolonged periods is *not* actually good for chronic back pain!**

Obviously, some rest is fine, and even necessary, but prolonged and extended periods of rest completely weaken the muscles. The muscles that are desperately needed to support the spine. Especially the lower spine. Have you ever noticed if you lie in bed too long, your lower back can get tight and sore? This is a pretty big indicator that your back needs more gentle movement to stay healthy.

The spine is doing a lot of work; the bones are intricate and need TLC. That is why walking is such a great medicine. It's a gentle movement that doesn't put too much strain on the back. But lying in one position for too long forces everything to cramp up.

Standing too long can do the same thing because all the muscles around the vertebrae are compressing on top of one another to cause pinching and less-than-optimal oxygen flow. Your muscles need to move and stretch to keep maximum levels of oxygen traveling through the blood.

Stretching sore muscles is another thing many of us tend to do. Especially those of us who like to get a lot of physical activity or lift weights. When the muscles get sore, we feel like we accomplished something. Some people even *enjoy* being sore. But then, our first impulse is to stretch the sore muscles to help "work out the knots." This is actually doing the opposite of what we want.

One of the reasons Yoga is so beneficial is because of the pose/counterpose symbiosis. A well-educated Yoga instructor always performs a counterpose for every posture they teach. But alas, as I have said, I have been to many classes where the teacher was clearly not well-trained and didn't seem to know any of this. They would do backbend after backbend after backbend and then end with something like a twist. Repeatedly doing backbends is fine, as long as you do several forward bends afterward (or in between) to counteract them.

When weightlifters go to the gym, they know not to work the same muscle group two days in a row. This tires out the muscles, but it's the same thing with stretching. If you stretch the same set of muscles, you need to extend the opposite set of muscles to counteract it. If you continue to target the same muscle groups without switching, they get worn out and loose while the opposite muscles get tight and atrophied. This is contradictory to what we want!

The best way to stretch your body if you have sore muscles is to extend the *opposite set of muscles*. For example, if your shoulder blades are sore, you need to stretch your chest. If your quads are sore, you need to stretch your hamstrings. The sore muscles need to rest, not be extended past their capacity when they are already overly exhausted.

Another prominent example of this would be the multitude of people I know [who suffer from back pain] who think they need to strengthen their back muscles. Now it is true that you want all of your muscles to be strong. That is for sure. But what is not going to help back pain is continuously trying to strengthen the back muscles. Especially if you're one of those people who uses those machines at the gym. You know the ones I'm talking about—the giant contraptions you sit on and look at the little pictures of the person that shows what area the machine targets on the body?

If your back is weak, you need to strengthen the *core muscles.* In all honesty, strengthening the core muscles will help protect every muscle in the body. But most importantly, because your back directly correlates to the backside of the core muscles, it is absolutely crucial the core becomes strong. If your core muscles are weak, your back muscles will overcompensate by stretching and pulling.

So while it is important to keep the back strong, the heavier focus should be on the core. Especially the lower abs and obliques. This is a huge game changer for many of my students. It amazes me how many people have ignored their cores for so many years. The other problem, is many people think they are strengthening their cores by doing simple exercises like crunches or sit-ups, which unfortunately, are outdated and downright risky. There are many ways to enhance the core muscles without doing these tedious and repetitive activities. Now, speaking of repetitive exercises, it's time for me to talk about...

REPETITIVE TRAUMA

I mention this because it is such a massive epidemic in today's society. And not just in America. Repetitive Trauma is running rampant everywhere. It comes from repetitive motions (even tiny ones) in our bodies which wreak havoc on our entire body's systems. It is also known as *Crossed Syndrome.* This reaction creates what you could call *fault lines,* which are basically areas of vulnerability inside the body. The result comes about due to muscular imbalances and postural distortions that pull the pelvis and spine entirely out of alignment over time. It is almost completely unavoidable in this day and age, which is why it is so prevalent.

BLOOD PRESSURE

If you have any issues with blood pressure, be very careful with how quickly you move from a reclining position to a standing position.

Rolling up one vertebra at a time from a forward bend isn't necessarily a good idea. Instead, bend the knees, straighten your back, and hinge up from the hips.

Be cautious with inversions. If you want to try being upside down, that's okay, just be very careful with it, and move slowly in and out of the positions. If you get a throbbing in your head every single time, that is a sign you need to do more preparations first.

Also, be careful about holding positions for too long. By moving our limbs into the different positions the Yoga postures entail, you cut off circulation to certain areas of the body while increasing it in others. This is called *vascular occlusion*. It affects the blood pressure in a negative way after a certain point.

If your blood pressure is already unbalanced, observe your body while you hold a posture. If you start to feel numbness or tingling at any time, that is your body telling you it is time to move out of the pose. Even if the teacher insists you hold it for another five breaths!

RESPIRATORY SYSTEM

Constricting the chest and throat area can be good for respiratory problems if done in very small quantities. Otherwise, only postures that open the front of the body are really safe to hold for more than 10 seconds. However, with continual practice, the lungs are likely to begin to repair themselves. As the respiratory problems dissipate, longer holds of these constricting postures can be experimented with.

JOINTS

Repetitive motions and heavy impact are usually the biggest contributors to joint problems. Therefore, "Yoga flow" classes can make joint problems worse in many cases. It is possible, if you spend enough time on alignment (such as in an *Iyengar* class), you will be able to guard your joints enough to protect them when you want to flow from one position to another.

But this requires more awareness than most of us are capable of.

Also, when suffering from any kind of joint problems, we should avoid jumping from one pose to another. Unless we can learn to make our bodies as light as a feather as we do it and land without making any kind of a thud!

SKELETAL STRUCTURE

When I worked with students, I noticed there were some particular things that just didn't quite work for them. So, because of my heavy interest in anatomy, I decided to figure out why.

In my Yoga teacher training, my teacher was also a registered nurse and an expert in human anatomy. She had been studying anatomy alongside Yoga for over 40 years. She pointed out that the muscles can stretch, but the bones cannot. This seems obvious, but many Yoga instructors try to force students into poses that just aren't safe for them. Poses their bodies will never be able to go into.

An example would be a pose like a squat. Some of us have ankle bones that literally hit the bones in our feet when we try to squat. No matter how much we practice squatting, no matter how flexible we become, we will never be able to change the fact that bone is hitting bone.

Therefore, a flat-footed squat will never be accessible to some people.

The bones in the pelvis and the bones in the shoulders or neck are good examples as well. Depending on how a certain human is built, once a bone is touching a bone, we have reached the end of our capacity for mobility. We will never be able to make our bones more flexible. And there is absolutely nothing wrong with that.

Muscles will be able to stretch, always increasing their flexibility, but bones are there to stay. So, try to figure out when you are attempting a posture if it is your skeleton tight muscles stopping you from going further. If it is just tight muscles, those muscles can be babied into eventually releasing all their tension. It may take a long time, but the process is called *proprioceptive neuromuscular facilitation*. This is a concept I have studied in-depth and will revisit in the next chapter.

NERVES AND MUSCLES

There are also limitations based around how individual muscles and nerves wrap around the bones. If the muscles are wrapped around a bone, and a nerve is caught in between them or vice versa, then it will cause shooting pain if specific positions are attempted.

For instance, to this day, I still can't comfortably touch my toes with my back straight and my feet together. This goes for standing or seated forward folds. But as soon as I separate my legs, I have no problem. After studying the human pelvis, as well as x-rays of my own pelvis, I learned there are certain nerves that pass through the pelvis that can get very inflamed if the muscles are too close to them. This is one of the reasons for debilitating sciatica.

Nerves can be very tricky. The human body is full of complicated networks and different channels and connections. I find the human nervous system to be the most fascinating of all the body systems, especially in the shoulders and hips and how they wrap around the bones and muscles. If you constantly or repeatedly pinch the nerve, numbness will result. It is possible this could eventually lead to permanent nerve damage in the affected area or even in neighboring areas of the body.

If you experience numbness or tingling in any part of your body when practicing a Yoga pose, this absolutely does not mean you should continue working on the same pose in the same way until the sensation goes away! It means you should ease out of the position enough that there is no numbness or tingling at all.

If the problem happens only when you repeat a series of poses over and over, it means the repetitive motion is causing inflammation in the muscles around the nerve and aggravating the nerve itself (Repetitive Trauma). Therefore, you should not be doing these repeated motions.

If the numbness and tingling only happen if you hold a pose for too long, then this simply means you should come out of the pose sooner.

You are the only one who can feel inside your body. Your teacher doesn't know what sensations are happening inside you. So, it is entirely up to you and your discretion to come out of a pose or sequence when you need to or to avoid it altogether.

INTERNAL VS. EXTERNAL ROTATION

Depending on which way our hips rotate naturally, forcing them to rotate the opposite way too often can actually lead to pinched nerves and other problems. Therefore, it is important we do not apply any of the Mindful Movement Techniques™ when in a position that accentuates an unnatural rotation of our hips.

There are only two categories here: internal rotators and external rotators. I am simply talking about the hips and pelvis. This may not seem like a very important thing to bring up, but knowing what type of rotation your body tends toward will help you understand why some poses are easier or harder for certain people.

So which one are you? It is easy to figure out.

When you sit on the floor, is it easier for you to sit with the bottoms of your feet together and your knees apart, or with your knees together and your feet apart?

The former means you are an external rotator; the latter means you are an internal rotator.

Neither of these is better than the other. It is just something to take into account when you practice Yoga. There are always exceptions to this, of course, but in general, men are more likely to be internal rotators, whereas women tend to be external rotators.

If you are an external rotator, certain poses will come much more naturally to you, such as cross-legged poses, wide-legged poses, or side bends. Basically, anything that requires the hips to open outward.

If you are an internal rotator, the poses that will come more naturally will be kneeling poses and backbends. Anything that draws your feet out and your knees in.

By all means, please feel free to practice any of the above poses as much as you like, just be sure not to push yourself too much when your hips are in an unnatural position for your type.

SCIATICA

This is another topic I could write an entire book about.

The reason I added it here is that *so many* people suffer from sciatica. And the interesting thing about this particular problem is that it can affect literally anyone at any point in life. So I decided it is worth noting. And it is possible to have it aggravated by—*gasp*—Yoga!

I won't get into a full breakdown on what exactly it is; there is enough information out there about it. But basically, the sciatic nerve runs all the way from your lower spine down your leg. On both sides. What tends to trigger sciatica is pressure on the nerve directly from inside the pelvis. This can come from a few different things; an injury–which changes the position of the muscles or the bones, inflammation–which makes the muscles swell and puts pressure on the nerve, or overstretching.

Once the sciatica pain is active (and believe me, you will know if it is or isn't), there are a lot of activities that aren't necessarily a good idea. One of the worst ideas is actually trying to stretch out the aggravated area. This is just going to exacerbate it more. I spent years doing Pigeon Pose (*Eka Pada Rajakapotasana*) when my sciatica was active because I wanted to stretch out the muscles around the nerve and open up the area. Turns out, this was having the *opposite* effect. All it did was stretch the tissue and the nerve over the ischial tuberosities (sitz bones) and just slow down healing.

Sciatica usually comes in flare-ups. It will flare up for a while, generally causing minor to excruciating pain, and then it will go back down. People with chronic sciatica (like I dealt with) spend more of their time dealing with flare-ups than not. Mine would usually act up with excruciating pain for two to three weeks at a time; then I would have a few days of peace before it acted up again.

There are two different types of flare-ups. The daily ups and downs, versus the long-term ups and downs. The daily flare-ups are somewhat deceptive because your sciatica is still *active*, you just can't feel it quite as much the whole day. There are points in the day where the pain peaks, and then it lessens for a little while; and it goes back and forth this way. This is because your pain receptors can't actually process that type of intense pain for a steady and consistent period of time. But don't be fooled—it is still active.

The long-term flare-ups would be what I was just talking about in the previous paragraph; you go for days or weeks of dealing with the sciatica pain every day. When the flare-up is over, you go for days or weeks (or hopefully months or years) at a time without feeling it at all. That means it is *not* active.

Now that I have learned how *not* to aggravate it, I have managed to keep it at bay. If I have a flare-up, it usually only lasts a day or two, and the pain is minor (or moderate at worst, if I really screw something up). And I go several months between flare-ups.

Here's the kicker though. You want to avoid most Yoga postures while in the middle of a flare-up. I didn't know this for a long time, and I forced myself through the Yoga postures even though the pain was horrible. I should have known better, but hey, you can learn from my mistakes at least, right?

Most Yoga sequences will aggravate sciatica. Things that make it worse are seated positions, forward bends, or anything that overly stretches the area around it, such as deep backbends, one-legged piriformis stretches (which are actually included as the best stretches to help sciatica in most literature you read about), or any kind of Sun Salutations (*Surya Namaskar*). So that's about 90 percent of the Yoga positions!

There is, however, a sequence I have designed specifically for people who deal with a sciatica flare-up. This is the *only* type of physical Yoga I do when my sciatica is active. I avoid everything else. And this is a form of a Moon Salutation (*Chandra Namaskar*).

If you are not familiar with a Moon Salutation, that's

okay; not a lot of people are—even in the Yoga-teaching community. But it is a flow of postures that all involve external rotation. And that is what you want when your sciatica is active. *External rotation.* Anything that turns the hips and legs out, because that releases the pressure of the muscles on the sciatic nerve itself.

So when my sciatica pain is really horrible, the only thing I can usually do is stand up and sway back and forth. Like an elephant. This gentle rocking motion eases the inflammation and helps keep the excessive pain at bay. I do Moon Salutations between the daily flare-ups.

There are several different types of Moon Salutations, so you have to be careful to make sure that all the sequences involve external rotation and no forward bends.

FIBROMYALGIA

This is yet another ridiculously broad topic.

Anyone who suffers from fibro-*anything* is a true warrior indeed! Fibromyalgia is a minimally understood condition that affects the muscular, nervous, and myofascial systems of the body. In basic terms, it means *constant pain everywhere*.

All. The. Time.

The tricky thing about this condition is that no one really knows what causes it or how to treat it.

But fibromyalgia is something I have had tremendous success with. Even though it only affects between 2 and 8 percent of the population, it seemed that these people were finding me in masses. I am a firm believer in the fact that you vibrationally attract the things to you that need you the most, or vice versa.

I also believe we vibrationally attract what we put out there, so, at the beginning of my healing career, I attracted a whole lot of whiners and complainers. Needless to say, I was a whiner and a complainer.

But now that I have shifted my perspective and approach, and raised my vibration, I attract people who are motivated and ready to heal. And both my students and I are tremendously more successful because of it.

As I started researching fibromyalgia more, I found it astounding that so many of these people were being completely ignored by health professionals and even loved ones. People just weren't taking this kind of pain seriously because they didn't understand it.

In all honesty, I believe it affects more than 8 percent of the population because I think a large number of cases go undiagnosed. The trick is that it doesn't usually fully set in until a person hits middle age. Very few people feel the effects from a young age—like I did.

But the anti-inflammation diet I put them on in my program, as well as the Mindful Movement Techniques™ have been unbelievably effective for the fibromyalgia sufferers I worked with. And it's a good thing, too, because right before my 30th birthday, when

I got my diagnosis, I was already carrying a full toolbox of knowledge with everything I needed to heal.

It didn't come as a particular shock to me. I was in pain everywhere all the time after all, and I knew it was very likely, considering my full-body arthritis issues as well (arthritis and fibromyalgia are frequently linked). So I didn't let it get me down. I was also very optimistic because I had been able to help so many other fibromyalgia sufferers. Now it was time to practice what I preached. Again.

The sad thing about this invisible illness is that so many people who suffer from it don't even know they have it. Or even if they do, no one around them believes that they're actually experiencing the amount of pain they truly are.

Believe me, I understand. To this day, there are very few people who understand the levels of pain I have come to be familiar with. So if you are one of the people who deal with this very unfortunate condition, I am here for you. I get you. I feel you. And I can help you.

Once again, I am not going to go into the full details of the origin or symptoms of fibromyalgia. I can save that for another book. But I do want to raise awareness about the subject. This condition is real. It is painful. And it is utterly impossible to explain to someone who has never experienced such a situation.

But I do want you to know there is hope. Yoga can do wonders and so can the dietary suggestions I make throughout this book. In fact, everything in this book can help tremendously with fibromyalgia.

One thing I do want to point out is that specific trigger points (I know for me it is my elbows, knees, and hips), can cause problems when doing some of the sequences. So please take care when following Yoga sequences because many postures can put direct pressure on some of these trigger points and cause tremendous pain.

Luckily, there is no known long-term damage, nerve damage, or any muscular damage caused by triggering these points on the body. But they *freaking hurt*! So no one wants to deal with that. Once again, hitting these trigger points will trigger the body's fight-or-flight responses and put you into a state of incredible anxiety. So let's avoid that.

Be very conscious of the trigger points and do everything you can to avoid applying pressure to these areas when practicing Yoga sequences. If that means you have to sit out certain postures, please do it!

MIGRAINES

I will keep this topic short and concise. When it comes to questions about Yoga postures while suffering from a migraine, the answer is ***don't***. Just don't. You do *not* want to do anything that will shift your heartbeat. Migraines usually come from an over-sensory stimulation, so you need to cut down all the senses around you. You need cool, dark, and quiet—with no strong smells. If you suffer from migraines, you probably already know this, though.

What you may not know, however, is that migraines usually come from an overgrowth of candida in the system as well as inflammation in the gut. I had heard this a few times but always brushed it off throughout my life. But no. This was legit. Cutting candida and inflammation out of your body will lessen your migraines significantly if not eradicate them altogether.

Migraine sufferers are usually just highly sensitive people. And I don't mean sensitive as in they cry at the drop of a hat, I mean sensitive as in bright lights, strong smells, loud noises, and weird textures affect them more than most people. *Sensory overload.* All coming from candida overgrowth and inflammation. Following the recommendations I lay out in the Anti-Yeast/Anti-Inflammation section will make a huge difference.

HYPERMOBILITY

Here, I am speaking especially to all the cheerleaders, gymnasts, acrobats, and ballet dancers who just love Yoga because it is so easy for them. As a former professional dancer, I fell into this category as well.

Though my arms and shoulders were never as flexible as I would have liked, I had such tremendous flexibility in my hips and legs that I relished every hip opener we did in class.

Every time the instructor suggested a pose that involved the hips and legs, I would sink into it as deeply as possible and just hang out there comfortably. Full split? Wide-legged forward bend? No problem! Stay there all day? Sure thing!

Then one day it all went wrong.

I was climbing Pikes Peak with a friend, and we had made it about 10 miles up, when I pulled my hip flexor. I was three miles from the top. Luckily, he was a pretty strong guy because he had to carry me most of the rest of the way!

The injury wasn't nearly as bad as it could have been. I was certainly very lucky. But it definitely affected my Yoga classes after that. I was suddenly unable to teach most of the poses I loved so much. So I had to start doing modifications of the postures.

The whole situation turned out to be a blessing in disguise because if this hadn't happened, I never would have learned this interesting tidbit about hyperextension:

There is such a thing as too flexible.

Some people hyperextend naturally, and some of us have developed excessive flexibility over the years. Flexibility is usually a very good thing, but only when it is also combined with equal strength.

If your muscles are only flexible and not strong, they are significantly more prone to pulling and tearing. This is what happened to me. I focused so much of my practice on increasing and sustaining my flexibility, I didn't pay enough attention to building up the muscles around it.

When it came time for a lunge, I would sink as deeply as I could into the position and then just hang out in it. Literally. I would allow the weight of my body to hang in the position instead of using the strength of my muscles to hold myself up. This turned out to be a major contributing factor to my severe inflammation and sciatica flare-ups.

And this is a pattern I see quite a lot, actually. Mostly in females, but in some men as well. Women tend to have a little more hip mobility, so they are more likely to make the mistake of allowing their flexibility to compensate for their lack of strength in those muscles.

My nurse friend told me that she sees this phenomenon a lot with hyper-flexible people. She said that she and her colleagues called it 'Yoga butt.' She used the analogy of taking a rope and rubbing it against the corner of a table. Eventually, the rope will start to fray, and finally break.

Now imagine your pelvis is the table, and your muscle is the rope. *Not a pretty thought.*

It is also an easy problem to remedy. It just requires kicking your ego to the side a bit. The way you do it is you don't go fully into the pose. You figure out how far your body can go, and then you ease up out of it about 50 percent at first, and then maybe only 20 percent with time.

You will quickly learn this actually makes the pose

more challenging. You are relying on the strength of your muscles to hold you in position instead of relaxing into it.

I actually had to spend about a year trying to *decrease* my flexibility. It took time, but it worked, and I was able to simultaneously build up the strength in the muscles I had over-stretched.

Now I am regaining a lot of that flexibility while maintaining my strength. This is where we can find balance.

But unless you have had some sort of injury like mine, there is no need to try to decrease your existing flexibility. Just focus on building up equal strength and resistance in those particular muscle groups in your flexible areas and not relying entirely on your flexibility.

A great way to build up strength in overly flexible muscle groups would be *static tension* and *vascular occlusion*. We will talk about what these terms mean in the next chapter.

METABOLIC RECONDITIONING

Now it's time to pat yourself on the back for making it this far. Because it's finally time to get down to the nitty-gritty. This part is all about reconditioning the physical body. But I felt it was essential to put the mental stuff as well as the internal cleansing stuff first because going through these things, in this particular order, makes everything that follows so much more effective.

The reconditioning methods would still be helpful without doing all the previous work, but I guarantee the results are astounding when you follow everything in the proper sequence.

For me, this is the fun part. I like to get out there and get my blood pumping, my heart racing, and break a good sweat. I love to feel my muscles burn and shake. But that is not the case for everyone. I get that. So don't be scared.

I promise these techniques can work for anyone. Including the quadriplegic friend I work with overseas. So just like everything else here, approach this with an open mind and the motivation to achieve transformational healing.

And just like at the beginning of this book, before I get into the *how,* I'm going to talk about the *why.* Why have I been rambling on for all these pages about cleaning the body and reconditioning your system?

Because I don't expect you to follow me blindly. If you do, that's cool, and your recovery will probably be smooth sailing and one of the easiest transformations out there. But most people are a lot more skeptical than that.

There are a couple of points I want to make here before I get into the actual techniques. The body's reconditioning takes place on a metabolic, hormonal, vascular, muscular, cellular, and neural level. Now that's a lot of levels.

Your metabolism does a whole lot more than just digest your food. When people think about the metabolism, they immediately jump to visions of eating more without gaining weight. It is commonly believed that people with high metabolisms digest their food more efficiently so they can stay thin and active. Whereas a person with a slow metabolism has a sluggish digestive system, therefore the fat goes through the body slower—absorbing into the tissues and making you put on weight like a hippo.

Neither of these things, however, is technically accurate. A fast or slow metabolism isn't the issue here. What the metabolism does is *regulate.* So, if you have a slow metabolism, it isn't necessarily a bad thing, but what you want is a *balanced* metabolism. An *active* metabolism. Fast isn't the answer. You want an overall *well-functioning* metabolism.

If you have a lot of pain in your body, or things just aren't working correctly—chances are your metabolism isn't either. Remember, *disease starts in the gut.* Now the metabolism and the gut aren't quite as linked as everyone thinks they are, but they are definitely interrelated. In fact, every body system is related to the gut. When your gut isn't functioning properly, nothing else in your body is. So we have to pay attention to these things.

The fastest way to get the gut running smoothly again is to reawaken the metabolism and start to recondition the metabolic processes. And yes, this does mean you will digest your food better. To do this, you have to activate certain levels of hormone production as well as trigger maximum oxygen flow and blood regulation. Sounds pretty fancy, huh? It's actually easier than it sounds. Let's start by talking about hormone balancing.

HORMONAL SOUP

People who have dealt with chronic pain for a long time have internalized the body's fight-or-flight reactions.

This puts the body in a state of hyperactive awareness. The average person's fight-or-flight response is only activated when the person becomes alarmed or scared. In some cases, like for those who are bipolar, the fight-or-flight response can also be activated during adrenaline rushes or increased bursts of serotonin when everything is feeling good.

But when your body is in so much pain for so long, it remains in a constant state of *fear*. Remember, **fear is just the anticipation of future pain**. When people are in pain, they clench up. They usually grit their teeth, make fists, and feel their stomachs tighten. But for people dealing with chronic pain . . . that doesn't go away. Sure, the clenching may lessen because one can't clench all the time, but the hormones that are triggered begin to plateau at higher levels than they would for the average person who doesn't deal with pain all the time.

All the stressors that are activated *remain* active, and eventually, we internalize them and bury them deep within our psyches. This is true on a physical and mental level, and of course, a spiritual level as well. This is one of the deeper-level reasons people with chronic pain deal with depression. It isn't just the surface-level reasoning for pain to make you depressed. It actually changes your body chemistry, and the longer you deal with it the deeper you bury it, and the more ingrained it becomes.

Now, the human body is incredible. It can handle an *awful* lot. But still, it can only handle so much for so long. Everything shifts eventually. There will always be that straw that breaks the camel's back. Things can build up for a long or short period before they finally break, the floodgates open, and s*** hits the fan.

Some of us have more than one shift like this in our lives. Sometimes it comes in the form of a mental breakdown, severe depression, or just a sudden feeling of hopelessness that doesn't go away. And for some, it's many little breakdowns instead of a few big ones. For me, it was definitely a few big ones. Things that went sour fast. Or at least that was how it seemed to me at the time.

But the truth was I had been internalizing so many things for so long without realizing it that it all just bubbled up to the surface one day. And then I realized how sick and messed up I truly was. The good thing about these types of experiences is that they help us learn and grow. Then we can actually look at them for what they really are—learning experiences.

This all comes back to hormonal reactions our bodies just can't regulate when they deal with so much pain for so long. This is why the reconditioning techniques are so crucial for regaining that hormonal balance. I like to call this mixed cocktail of hormones the ***hormonal soup***. When all the ingredients are mixed correctly, and then heated up all at once, magnificent things can happen! But how we trigger the reconditioning in our body can make the difference between a can of soup concentrate heated in the microwave or a

55-ingredient gourmet bisque prepared over an open flame with care. Okay. Maybe my metaphors are overly complex...

Anyhoo, there is a way to reactivate the hormonal and metabolic activities in the body to regulate and support each other. Once this happens, the body's ability to heal itself increases at a rapid rate. You will start to notice improvements almost immediately.

These systems in our bodies that have been dormant for so long are just waiting to be reawakened, and when that happens, all sorts of things will shift, not only on the physical level but the mental and spiritual levels as well. Thought processes become clear, emotions stabilize, and a sense of peace and tranquility increases.

Another vital factor to keep in mind here is that a cross-pattern motion of the body's limbs is essential for the hypothalamus, pituitary, and brain hemisphere balancing.

"Brain Gyms" have been exploding in popularity for this exact reason. If you aren't familiar with a Brain Gym, it is a series of mental exercises that help to trigger both hemispheres of the brain to keep your cognitive functions at optimal levels. They are frequently used by psychiatrists, therapists, and anyone dealing with people suffering from mental illnesses. Especially Autism. But that isn't all the brain does.

The brain directly correlates to our physical health as well. Have you ever noticed you get brain fog when you are constipated? When your body is full of toxins, and they are all just sitting there having a party in your system, this affects everything from your nervous system to your skeleton. You want to be firing on all cylinders all the time, but how can you when you can barely even get the vehicle to start?

As we go further into the Mindful Movement Techniques™, the cross-motion patterns here will come into play as well as the metabolic reconditioning. The interesting part about this is that all this takes place completely naturally when we walk. The arms are swinging, the legs are swinging, and everything is happening in a series of beautiful fluid movements.

Unless they're not.

When your body is so toxic, walking just doesn't cut it anymore because, frankly, it's just not enough. And you may not even be walking properly either. People who suffer from chronic pain actually tend to have less arm movement when they walk. It has been said that this is because the person is always in a clenched-up and fearful position from the pain, but a lot of this has to do with the misfiring in the brain hemispheres as well.

When it comes to chronic pain, most of us can probably forget about running! But this particular series of motions explains why marathon runners get such a "runner's high." Especially the cross-country runners who do it for long stretches at a time. The longer you put your body in this state, the more hormones kick into gear, and the more everything starts to realign. But

I'm not saying you should go out and start training for a marathon; running isn't even ideal for everyone, and it is *almost* never suitable for a chronic-pain sufferer. Believe me. I would know. I still mourn my running career to this day.

But if running is something you have done in the past, or still want to do, there is hope. It's just a matter of taking care of your body as you do it. Which we are going to go into here. The main thing is setting aside the ego long enough to let your body rest. Because when you have autonomy to control when you rest, your body will actually work harder. I will explain this further when I cover the *Repetitive Resting Technique.*

So without further ado, let's get into the Mindful Movement Techniques™.

THE MINDFUL MOVEMENT TECHNIQUES™

Now, if you read *Yoga for You,* then you are already somewhat familiar with these techniques. I talked about them somewhat, but for chronic pain sufferers, they have been restructured to a degree. The basic concept is the same, but the execution is a little different. Instead of trying to cater each Yoga posture and sequence to our individual needs, we are specifically trying to trigger the body's natural ability to overcome pain.

The techniques are geared toward increasing flexibility and strength simultaneously. It is imperative we find a synergistic balance between the two. I strongly urge you to learn them one at a time, *in order!* When you feel you are comfortable with the techniques, you can begin to interchange them, and apply them to other areas of your life as well.

The Mindful Movement Techniques™ are designed to be done for 20 minutes, three times weekly. Now, you have to admit that is not a huge time commitment. Of course, you can do more, but you don't want to overdo it. So, just remember to move forward with baby steps. You can also apply these techniques to other activities. You can do them at your regular Yoga classes or even use some of the concepts while you're walking the dog.

TECHNIQUE #1

Breathe and Sink

This involves proper adaptation of *Proprioceptive Neuromuscular Facilitation* (PNF).

Yes, I know—big words!

This is the scientific backing for why it is necessary to practice Yoga at least twice per week. PNF is what triggers a muscle to relax and release. When PNF is properly activated, it lasts for up to 72 hours. Meaning, when you trigger that amount of flexibility in your muscle, it will remain that flexible for up to 72 hours.

When practiced, the results are pretty astonishing. It will increase your flexibility to a remarkable degree in a very short amount of time. This extra flexibility will continue to rapidly increase as long as you are diligent about practicing two to three times per week.

This process tricks the muscles into relaxing and then, in turn, releasing. If your muscles can relax long enough to allow oxygen to integrate and start to flow, then they can safely allow the flexibility to increase every time.

Now, when we practice our physical Yoga postures, we are practicing many forms of PNF using our own body weight. If you have done the math in your head, you now understand why it is important to practice Yoga at least twice per week. The increase in flexibility lasts for 72 hours, so you need to utilize PNF by doing Yoga at least every 72 hours (broken record here, I know). That is how you will rapidly gain and maintain the flexibility in your muscles.

The best way to consciously apply PNF through your Yoga practice is to make sure to sink a little deeper into each pose with each exhalation.

For example, when you find yourself in a twist, breathe as deeply as possible and try to sink deeper into the twist every time you exhale. Allow your body weight to take over and pull your body deeper and deeper as time goes on. The longer you hold, the more flexibility you will gain.

When we move between stagnant positions, we should exhale. The inhalation is for the stagnant position itself. Exhalation helps us to move fluidly from one posture to the next. It is apparent when you practice any sort of Yoga posture or stretch that you can move deeper into that stretch as you exhale. This is because the exhalation allows the body to be free from tension for just a moment.

This is another reason we need to learn to deepen

our practice with time. If we continue doing Yoga the same way after 10 years, as we did for the first 10 days, we will never make any progress. This is why a mindful approach is so important to the learning process.

For another example, if you are in a forward bend, every time you exhale, allow the weight of your body to make your torso sink even closer to your legs. The longer you hold a pose, the closer your torso will get to your legs, and the more you are going to get out of it.

Now PNF is more difficult to apply to some poses (such as push-up positions or standing postures). But it is possible if you use mindfulness to observe which muscles are actually activated when you practice them. This comes with practice and observance.

If this seems like too much for you, don't worry. Just use this technique when you do poses that focus on stretching more than strengthening. Like a seated forward fold, side bend, or twist. You want to safely increase your flexibility without over-stretching the muscles and causing them to be strained and flimsy.

Hot Yoga can speed up this process quite a bit. But we also need to be careful not to soften up the muscles or the ligaments to the point where we can pull them. This is actually how pregnant women can damage themselves because, during pregnancy, women's ligaments become more malleable. This leads to increased flexibility but also increased risk of injury. Also, warming up the muscles too much can lead to inflammation and deterioration of the tissue if the muscles don't already have a strong foundation of freely flowing oxygen and decent blood flow.

But as long as you mindfully and consciously practice PNF during a hot Yoga class, then you will avoid injury due to over-stretching and over-warming.

My primary goal is to teach people how to properly take care of their bodies. To help them understand that their forms are unique, and then learn to adjust their attitudes and physical practices accordingly.

Another helpful benefit of PNF is that it breaks up buildups of connective tissue because it will require you to hold the poses longer. If you are at home practicing alone on your mat, or in front of a DVD, you can simply pause in each of the seated or reclining poses. Stay there for a minimum of 10 to 25 breaths. With each exhalation, see if you can stretch a little bit deeper into the pose.

I am now going to share with you the connective tissue story I tell all my students at some point in our time together. The teacher in my Yoga Anatomy training course called a buildup of connective tissue "The Fuzz."

Every night when you sleep, or whenever your body isn't mobile for that matter, your muscles and joints begin to develop a thin layer of the Fuzz. This is a white, sticky material that does indeed look quite fuzzy. It is really called connective tissue.

When you wake up in the morning, you stretch yourself out and begin to move around. This breaks up the Fuzz that has built up in your body overnight. The Fuzz is always developing, but if you make a continuous effort to break it apart, all that will remain is a thin layer.

However, if you don't make a continuous effort to break up the Fuzz, it will begin to build up. It will build layer upon layer as if you were adding multiple coats of paint to a surface.

As the layers build up, they become less malleable and begin to calcify. The Fuzz becomes tougher and tougher, and eventually, even hard. Once it reaches this state, it becomes significantly more difficult to break apart.

It is similar to maintaining dental hygiene, where the plaque that builds up on your teeth daily eventually becomes tartar if it is neglected.

If you want to avoid having connective tissue buildup, you need to make sure you allow oxygen to flow into your muscles (too much connective tissue can suffocate the muscle, leading to muscle atrophy). This is where Yoga comes in.

Now the secret to avoiding this is very simple: *move!*

Moving and stretching breaks up the Fuzz. If you break it up every day, it won't build up! Therefore, it won't calcify.

But what if this has already started to happen?

Don't worry. It is still reversible. This technique is extremely effective for breaking up a buildup of calcified connective tissue as well as increasing flexibility.

This is because you hold the postures for so long. Traditionally, in styles such as *Yin Yoga,* you hold a pose for no less than five minutes, and sometimes as long as 30 minutes!

When you hold a posture for this long, PNF naturally takes place. But it is always a good idea to be conscious of PNF while doing so. This helps the process along.

TECHNIQUE #2

Repetitive Resting

Remember when we talked about Repetitive Trauma earlier? How tiny repetitive motions can have big consequences later on down the road? This is kind of the opposite.

This is also where I get to tell you that there is such a thing as *too much exercise.*

Exercising too frequently, or too intensively, actually weakens the immune system as well as the metabolism.

For good health, we need a good, strong metabolism. A well-functioning and high-performing metabolism.

As mentioned earlier, this doesn't always mean we want to *speed up* the metabolism, and there are even people out there who believe we need to slow it down, but what we really want is a properly *balanced* metabolism.

For proper balancing, we need to know when to stop. When we are pushing ourselves too hard.

Now, this is going to be different for everyone. Some people can go a lot longer and harder than others, depending on their constitution. For instance, in Ayurveda, Vata-types tend to tire quickly and easily. Whereas Kapha-types can go long and steady without tiring at all.

Just remember there is nothing wrong with that. It doesn't mean you aren't healthy, it just means you are different from the person next to you.

Just remember: *When you get hot and breathless, stop and rest.*

That's right. I said *stop and rest.*

This isn't a book about training to run a marathon. This isn't a book about endurance sports. This is a book about reconditioning your body, mind, and spirit to overcome chronic pain through Yoga.

When we get too hot and breathless, we tend to get sloppy in what we are doing. Maybe the push-ups have gotten so hard we are letting our hips sag. Maybe that lunge position might not look perfect, but hey, at least we are still doing it, right?

Not so much.

When we push ourselves too hard, we begin to lose that self-awareness that makes Yoga so beneficial. Remember how I said that repeatedly doing a Yoga posture incorrectly can work against your favor? I also talked about how every pose needs to be followed by a counterpose—well, this technique is like the counterpose to Repetitive Trauma. It is vital that we remain completely aware of our bodies when we do this.

There is nothing wrong with pushing ourselves. It is good to push. But if you push to the point of exhaustion, stop. Take a break. Rest. Breathe. Wiggle around. Then get right back into it.

Ideally, we will push until we can push no more, and then rest until we feel renewed and ready to start again with total enthusiasm.

But the amount of time we rest is going to be different for everyone. I tend to take fewer but longer breaks when I push myself. This works very well for me, and I know that. But I know others who take many short breaks, and that is what works for them.

I like to see my students take multiple breaks when I push them really hard. And I encourage them to take as many breaks as they need for as long as they need.

This is what helps the body reset and prepare for the upcoming exertion.

By avoiding over-exhaustion, we build up tolerance and stamina. This, in turn, strengthens not only our muscles, but our nervous systems, circulatory systems, and of course, metabolisms.

TECHNIQUE #3
Pressurized Pulsing

Excess post-exercise oxygen consumption - EPOC

This is where we get that breathing going heavy. It's where we build up all of that heat inside the body to get us breathless to the point where we have to rest. But we still want to do it *gently*.

We are not going to start running up and down flights of stairs or doing jumping jacks until we see sparkles. We are going to do gentle movements repeatedly for an extended period. When your body gets tired, you will know. And like I just explained, that's when you rest.

This particular technique involves a rapid pulsing motion over some regions of the body which build up pressure in that targeted area. This does get some of the vascular occlusion going, but most importantly, we are building heat and pressure. Once pressure has accumulated to the point where you can't keep going—stop and rest.

This technique goes hand-in-hand with the *Repetitive Resting Technique,* as you can see.

This is the ultimate technique for making you feel the burn! It's also a key contributing factor to a healthy production of human growth hormone (HGH) which is crucial for keeping your muscles healthy.

Aside from the tremendous benefits for reconditioning the hormonal cocktail happening within your body (which balances your body's adrenaline and serotonin responses as well as the production of endorphins which are necessary to handle pain), there are some added benefits as well. These hormone-producing actions are also skin-tightening, muscle-toning, fat-burning, and endurance-building.

Sounds pretty appealing, right?

This technique is also super easy to do, but I'm not even going to pretend like it doesn't start to suck after a hot minute! The instructions are simple: extend yourself into a posture . . . and pulse. Keep pulsing until you can pulse no more.

The most uncomplicated introduction to this technique is to simply bring your arms out to the sides, parallel to the ground. Now begin to pulse those arms up and down or in tiny circles. They're not moving too much, you're only moving them about an inch or two up and down at a time, but keep going.

You will start to feel the burn very quickly. If you

want to push yourself a bit, and if this is easy for you, lower yourself down into a squat position. Keep pulsing those arms.

If you want to push a little bit further, then make fists with the hands and tighten up the arms all the way into the shoulder blades while you pulse. Try to keep your face and the rest of your body relaxed, though.

Push as long as you can; you will know when you need to stop. Believe me. Just remember to rest as long as you need to, and then hop right back into it with full force.

Like the other techniques, this can be done with any area of the body. But only do one area at a time because your body isn't actually capable of multitasking. You need to give your full attention to *one area at a time* only. If you want to target your butt and thighs, lower down into a squat, but keep your hands together in prayer position this time while you pulse only your hips up and down. Same concept.

You can do this with leg lifts, twists, and even push-ups. The pulsing push-up is fun if you like a good challenge! Come to a high push-up position, then tuck your elbows in as close to your body as possible, lower yourself down about an inch from the ground, and then pulse. You might need to take more than a few breaks!

Don't forget to breathe!

TECHNIQUE #4

Press and Squeeze

I can't stress enough just how important it is to build up your strength along with your flexibility. We need to spend equal time on both. Strength and flexibility support and build on one another. I have seen wild improvements in an individual's ability to burn fat and calories in addition to building muscle when this technique is utilized correctly.

The technique consists of tightening and squeezing the muscles to restrict blood flow to certain areas of the body. This involves *static tension* and *vascular occlusion*. Static tension is the tightening and vascular occlusion is the restriction of blood flow.

Now, if you know anything about these terms already, there might be an alarm going off in your head telling you these are actually *bad* things, which can certainly be true if done excessively, involuntarily, or improperly.

But if you use these concepts in a mindful way, they can actually be very beneficial for strengthening your muscles and skeleton, as well as your nervous system and cardiovascular system.

Static tension is usually taking place when you are working very hard in a pose, but from an outside perspective, it doesn't look like you are doing anything at all. Usually, the person is standing completely still but applying great force to the internal body.

A starting point I use with my students is usually having them put both of their palms together in a prayer position. Then I have them press their palms together firmly. From the outside, it may not look like anything has changed, but for the person doing this, a tremendous effort is being put forth.

You can apply this to literally any position. It's just a matter of tensing up a muscle group and then letting it go. To achieve a safe level of vascular occlusion—the kind that begins to stimulate hormone production—the trick is to start small and work your way up. Then do this in repetitions.

- Try holding your arms out in front of you, parallel to the floor.
- Inhale deeply, and at the top of the inhalation, tighten up those arms and shoulders, making fists with your hands. Really squeeze.
- Hold this tightness for one second and then release.

- Now do the same thing, but hold for two seconds.
- Release.
- Repeat, but hold for three seconds.
- Release.
- Then four seconds...
- ...then five seconds...

After you have become very experienced with this technique, you can work your way up to 10 seconds. Otherwise, just repeat the process over and over; working your way up from one to five seconds. Then start over again at one.

Try this in all the different muscle groups in the body. The legs, hips, glutes, abdominals, chest, even the neck and face. I even start some people with this when they are lying down because it is easier to keep the rest of the body relaxed when we are lying down.

You want to restrict the blood flow just enough to get it pumping more actively during the release. This, in turn, will bring more circulation to the area as well as begin to produce a healthy hormonal response.

With time and repeated practice, you will notice an improvement in your stamina. Your circulation will also become more efficient, improving blood flow to all areas of the body, including the brain. This will also increase mental productivity and give you more clarity overall.

Most importantly, utilizing this technique will

condition your metabolism. And remember what I talked about earlier? Both disease and health start in the gut!

NOW LET'S KEEP THE BRAIN HEALTHY

MENTAL CLARITY

Meditation has been proven to improve concentration, focus, memory, and comprehension. But many people don't even know where to start. Some do not even realize that they have already started a meditation practice because don't know how to develop it yet.

Should you meditate?

There is really no quick or easy answer to this.

Meditation is going to be different for everyone. Chances are, there is already something in your life that could be considered meditation.

Meditation doesn't always have to be sitting on a cushion with your back straight and your eyes closed while you sit quietly for hours without moving.

Although I still enjoy sitting on the floor to meditate, I go about it in multiple other ways as well.

I bring my meditation into my Yoga practice. I meditate while I hike and run. I meditate while I cook, while I do dishes, and while I shower. This has become easier for me over the years.

Anyone can meditate.

And everyone, just like with a physical Yoga practice, has a practice that will be unique to them and most beneficial for their own personal types.

Your personal type will also change over time. Maybe now you can only meditate while you walk the dog, but in a few years, perhaps you will much prefer to meditate in silence, before the sun comes up, in a seated position with your eyes closed.

Many enlightened masters are never seen in a traditional meditation posture. Their meditation is their life. Their work. Their message.

My current teacher said that serving others was the only meditation I needed. Once I took this principle into action, I started to find myself in deep states of meditation even when I wasn't planning on it.

It was my ego telling me I needed to sit down to meditate. But eventually, my heart was able to override my ego and tell me that all I needed to do was be selfless. To learn to love and serve others was all it took to make that final leap I had been trying to make for so long. I am not saying I am perfect in any way. Far from it! But reaching an acceptance of where we are in life is the first step toward allowing ourselves to move forward.

FOCUSING THE MIND

Maybe a traditional meditation practice is what you need. Or maybe all you need to move forward is to just approach your daily activities with a little more mindfulness. Sometimes that is plenty.

Through mindfulness and meditation, we can begin to work our way through life with more focus and clarity. Things will become easier for us. We will be able to think better, to be kinder and more loving.

We can step up to situations with confidence that perhaps we would have shirked away from in the past.

Ancient wisdom says the only true path to satisfaction is to let go of all desires. Only when we have no desires are we truly free from wanting.

Look around you. Look within. How much of this could you do without?

I am asking this not only on a physical level but an emotional level as well. The baggage we carry around is weighing us down, and if we can release it, we will be able to fly!

While this will perhaps be a work in progress for the

rest of my life, I am grateful for every step I take to get there. Even the steps backward.

This may be my own unique journey, but it is certainly not unusual. Everyone has to find their own path. The only way to do it is to keep trying and to be gentle with ourselves. Remember, things are never going to unfold the way we expect them to. Which is why I want to talk about this next subject.

CHRONIC PAIN WHILE TRAVELING

I know quite a bit about this particular subject because I travel so much. Having dealt with chronic pain my entire life, and also being nomadic, has presented an interesting array of challenges.

Many people who suffer from chronic pain are completely terrified to travel because they don't want their pain to act up and ruin their good time. I understand this to an extent, but I never let it stop me. Sometimes, looking back, I think maybe it should have. But hey, if I hadn't had such a terrible flare-up in India, and ended up in the emergency room, I never would have had that epiphany that transformed everything for me.

But I do want to let you know there is hope. There are definitely some things you can do to avoid or minimize pain flare-ups while you travel. I find this is particularly important to note because even for those of us who can say we have overcome chronic pain, we may still occasionally have some issues with it from time to time throughout our lives. But everybody does. Every single person on this entire planet has and will experience pain during their lifetimes. There is no avoiding it. But we can choose whether or not we *suffer*. I truly believe that.

The thing about traveling is that not only is it very inconvenient to have pain flare-ups during your travels, but traveling is frequently the *cause* of these flare-ups. There are so many factors here.

If you're sitting in a car on a long road trip, you're scrunched up in one position, and if you're the one driving, you're just repeatedly using the muscles in your feet to work the pedal. You also have to grip the steering wheel, stare continuously at the road, and chances are (if you are a good driver and you focus on the road properly), you are not being very mindful of what your body is doing.

If you travel by air, the same issues with scrunching up in the seat are there, but on top of that, there is trying to sleep with your neck all sideways, while avoiding leaning over on the person next to you, and then the altitude alone creates a whole slew of problems!

And if you bring baggage, if it has wheels, you have to lean sideways all awkwardly and unevenly to drag that bag with you, or if you carry a backpack (which is my personal preference), that is another weight on your back. The worst possible contender is carrying a heavy duffle-bag on one shoulder.

And then there is the food problem. If you change time-zones, not only did this mess up your circadian rhythm but your digestive tract needs regularity. It's utterly impossible to do when you travel because you have no control of getting your meals at convenient times, especially if the time itself is what is changing! On top of that, it is also challenging to find healthy options that are ideal for digestion.

With all that being said, here are some things you can do to counteract this:

ACIDITY AND AIR TRAVEL

First of all, I said traveling by airplane makes you very acidic. Just being up in that altitude alone dehydrates your body and shocks your system into becoming less alkaline. I tend to get horrible migraines when I fly, and shortly after, the sciatica likes to kick in because I allowed my muscles to get so dehydrated.

The best way I know to alleviate this is to drink hot water (I know, big surprise). Drink one to three cups of hot water before you get on the airplane, and then at least one to three after you land. This hydrates your colon better than anything, and this will help to keep you more alkaline.

I know that some people don't like to get up and go to the bathroom a lot on planes, especially if you're in a window seat, but the people next to you can deal with it. Your health is more important than his or her temporary convenience. If I could convince the people sitting next to you to drink the hot water as well, I certainly would!

I also like to bring mineral supplements with me on airplanes. Even though I am generally not a supplement advocate, good quality minerals have treated me very well on airplane adventures. There is no real way to avoid getting more acidic on an airplane, but keeping your body appropriately hydrated does alkalize your system enough to prevent severe flare-ups. Especially if you are a migraine sufferer.

As I also said, I prefer to carry a backpack. I am also cautious when I pack the bag to make sure I am distributing the weight evenly on both sides of it. And I try to put all the heaviest weight toward the back of the bag, so it is the closest to my spine. The closer the weight is to your core, the easier your body can counteract it.

I am very conscious when I pick up the backpack to try to switch back and forth between which arm I pick it up with and swing it onto my shoulder. Tiny motions like this can throw everything out of whack if done unconsciously. The same with the rolling suitcase. Try to switch which hand you pull the suitcase with as you walk. Again, these movements may seem very slight, but if you keep doing it, it can change your interspinales muscles just enough to cause spinal discomfort and inflammation.

For road trips, I highly recommend stopping as much as possible to get out and stretch your legs. I Like to swing my arms back and forth in front of one another—switching which arm goes on top each time—this is that brain-hemisphere-crossing thing I was talking about. This is also fantastic for getting your blood moving.

You need to keep your brain super clear; especially if you are the one driving. You need to be able to stay focused. On top of that, you need the oxygen and the blood moving throughout your body because you're sitting it in a stagnant position for long stretches at a time. Just stretch and move as much as possible. If you can tolerate stopping every hour, please do.

The trickiest part about travel is *food.* There are lots of people who have written books and teach classes on this subject. *How to eat healthy while you travel.* But the thing is, healthy is different for everyone. So all I can really say on this issue is *just try to stay alkaline.* Hot water, hot water, hot water! You can stop at gas stations and get *hot water!* Any restaurant you go to—you can order *hot water!* Yes, sometimes this might annoy the server, so just don't stiff him or her on the tip!

The obvious answer I hear the most is just to bring your own food, but this isn't always easy or possible. Plus, depending on how long you travel for, you obviously run out of the food! And when you travel through third-world countries, stopping at a nearby Whole Foods isn't an option. I do try to bring snacks with me, but because the most digestible foods are not things you can travel with very easily, it requires you to just get downright creative and resourceful.

There's no way around it really, just try to keep everything else in your body as alkaline as possible.

Did I mention hot water?

After discussing such situational pain, I am going to move into another—rather delicate—subject. However, it is a particular situation we will *all* experience. Please approach this next chapter with an open mind.

END-OF-LIFE PAIN

This is another subject that is near and dear to my heart. Probably more so than anything else I have mentioned in this book. Although I can relate the most to those who suffer from chronic pain, because I have been there, I have had a lifelong passion for the dying process.

I have included terminal illness here because it is closely related to chronic illness and chronic pain (and for some, it is directly related). It is no secret that most people who are preparing for the dying process are dealing with pain as well. Unfortunately, the majority of people on this planet meet their demise from some kind of terminal illness. According to the World Health Organization, nine of the top 10 causes of death worldwide are some variation of terminal illness.

In my years working with hospice patients, I have seen many transitions. It is beautiful on so many levels.

The transition itself is always an honor to witness, but the time leading up to that transition is usually the part that most people fear. The pain. Death and suffering do not *have* to go hand in hand, but it will if we let it.

The most important part is to learn to let go of the fear. Many people approach the end of their lives with a lot of fear, but from what I have seen, even the most fearful people still have a tremendous sense of peace when the transition itself actually happens. And in cases such as hospice or palliative care, I believe that avoiding painkiller usage has been rendered completely unnecessary. There is no need to suffer through physical pain if you don't have to.

This brings me back to sorting out your priorities. At the end of life, where do you think your priorities will be? There is a point with a diagnosis of a terminal illness where the idea of death goes from being distant, to very real, to present moment—here and now. Some people are diagnosed with terminal diseases and then end up making a full recovery and live for 30–50 more years. There are others who remain terminal for longer than expected, living another five or 10 years. And then there are those who *know* it is coming. They must accept their fates. This isn't a matter of just giving up, but it's a matter of accepting what the universe brings you.

There is nothing wrong with accepting your death and your mortality. These are completely natural events that every single one of us are going to have to go through eventually.

So when you know that you are truly terminal, when the end is coming soon, and there is no avoiding it, and you have reached a point of acceptance with it, your priorities are going to shift.

There is no longer any reason to worry about repairing the physical body. It is time to accept that we need to let the body go. There might even be a point where we need to accept that the mind is fading as well. This is perfectly natural and part of the dying process. The only thing left to recondition at this point is the soul. Nourish your soul until your dying breath.

However, even with the best pain medication out there, such as morphine, there are still instances where pain is experienced.

For instance, my father recently passed away from cancer. I sat with him while it happened. I went and stayed with my family for the three months leading up to his final transition. I stayed at his bedside and did my best to take care of him through the entire process.

It was actually very beautiful to watch. From the moment he knew there was no turning around, he accepted his fate with grace. He made an effort to take care of the things he wanted to do, see the people he wanted to see, and prepare for his transition. He had no fear.

But he did have pain. A lot of pain. That was by far the hardest to watch.

What was so interesting about my father was where he set his priorities. He didn't like the way the morphine or all the other drugs affected his mental faculties. So he opted out of them completely! He wanted to stay alert and keep his memory; he was still holding on to life a little bit. But there was a point where something in him shifted.

I believe it was after he felt he had handled everything he needed to, he had seen everyone he wanted to, and he was ready to just lay back and let the transition happen. That was the point where he became complacent about the painkillers. He accepted his morphine in larger and larger doses. He knew it was time to let everything go. I can only imagine what his soul was experiencing at the time. I'm sure it was incredible!

As I sat with him, I would watch his eyes flutter; he would stare off calmly. It was such an honor to be present for so much of that experience; his eyes would dart back and forth, he would talk to someone the rest of us couldn't see, he would check his watch all the time and talk about needing to go somewhere. He was getting ready for a journey. A journey he was looking forward to.

He was in and out of being coherent the very last few days. And a day or two before his final breath, he made some closing statements—as if he were on stage and the curtains were about to close. Then he went to sleep, and he didn't speak again. That was it.

You feel so helpless when you watch someone else suffer. The way I would feel helpless when I would watch my daughter suffer, or when I happened to pass by a snake lying in the road recently that had been run over and was just slowly suffering to death. It's a different kind of helpless than the helplessness you experience when dealing with your *own* pain.

When it's *your* pain, you feel like a *victim*; you wish you could do anything to make it end. But when you see someone else suffering, especially if you have experienced true pain for yourself, you can empathize with them and wish you could free them from their pain.

This is one of those things that makes the dying process so beautiful. ***The anticipation of freedom.*** I think this is why people, at the end of their lives, have significantly less fear. It decreases as they get closer to their final transition. Like I said, *fear is the anticipation of future pain.* But when you are already dealing with pain, and you know the end is coming, the fear begins to dissipate because you know you don't have to worry about it in the future.

My dad looked forward to his death. Not in a morbid way, but in a very free kind of way. I talked with him a lot up until his final days. He said he didn't have any regrets. Of course, there were some things he might have done differently if he could do it again, but all in all, he was very pleased with the way his life had unfolded.

He was ready to go. And I was ready to see him go. I was happy for him when he finally passed. I smiled as his soul and his body parted ways. I still smile to think about where he is and what he's doing now. Don't get me wrong, I was still sad, and I did cry. But the sadness that comes from losing a loved one is really just our own selfishness. We are sad because we are the ones left behind. The transition for the person dying is different, and it can be joyful.

It is unnecessary to burden them with our own grief and suffering. That is for us to deal with.

So we should be happy for them! This is a powerful way to show them love and the deepest consideration.

ALLOWING THE TRANSFORMATION TO HAPPEN

Some people have completely settled into their pain and suffering. They are actually **comfortable in their discomfort.** They use it as a reason for whining or getting sympathy. Some even become so dependent on the illness that it is eventually all they know. They identify with it, and it becomes part of their ego-self.

Some people just like the attention. I think a lot of us have been this way to an extent. I know I have. But getting out of this mindset is so important because it's the only way we can truly break free from the cycle. The *chronic pain cycle.*

I won't give a lecture here about becoming more disciplined. Discipline isn't the issue here; it's a matter of figuring out what you want and how bad you want it. If you want to ultimately overcome your chronic pain, what steps are you willing to take to do that?

There is no need to go on a ridiculously restrictive

diet for the rest of your life. Believe me. I did this for years. I would even jokingly tell people the only things I could eat were grass and dirt. But this got me nowhere, other than miserable and feeling like I was missing out on things.

It isn't necessary to purify your body to the point that the slightest exposure to any kind of toxin will send it spiraling out of control. I have a friend who has raised her child on such a clean, healthy diet that the child can't even eat a piece of Halloween candy without being sick for a week.

Taking things to this extreme just puts the body even further out of balance. And if we are already dealing with chronic pain, we are already out of balance. We need to have a somewhat resilient system to combat everything going on around us in life. We can never be 100-percent toxin-free because just daily life and the world in general, throws toxins at us all the time. But if we can recondition our bodies to handle these toxins, we can heal and move forward in our lives.

This doesn't mean we should eat cake, ice cream, and hot dogs all the time. There are certain things you eat that you will be immediately aware of the fact they aren't good for you. This happens especially as your mindfulness increases.

When I go places where I am surrounded by delicious temptations (I'm not going to lie, donuts are my biggest weakness), the people with me are always amazed that I have so much self-control. People always ask how I can handle life without sugar or something of the like. My response to this is: "If every time you ate an ice cream cone, somebody smashed your hand with a hammer, you probably wouldn't eat any more ice cream cones, right?"

Inevitably, the answer is always yes. Your brain makes the association with the negative effect. Therefore, you stop wanting to do that thing because you know you won't even be able to enjoy it.

Nowadays, it is like that for me with certain foods. I know if I eat something with high fructose corn syrup or MSG I immediately start to get a migraine. The same goes for certain foods that cause immediate gut-wrenching pain.

The reason so many people continue with bad habits, especially food habits (but I'm not just talking about food here, this can apply to physical mannerisms or even emotional habits), is because the consequence is *indirect.*

We know if we eat a gallon of ice cream every day for a year, we are going to get fat. But the fat comes on slowly. We look in the mirror each day and don't necessarily notice the weight gain until the change is more drastic. If you ate a gallon of ice cream, and then immediately looked in the mirror and saw yourself 50 pounds heavier, that would be a very *direct* consequence! When the consequence is that immediate, we are less likely to indulge in something we know is not good for us.

As you build your self-awareness, you will feel immediately and directly if something isn't conducive to your overall well-being. I have become very hyper-aware of extremely negative people, chaotic environments, music, activities, and food that lower my vibration. I can feel it almost instantaneously. This keeps me from wanting to indulge in these things now.

Some may call this a curse, but I call it a blessing.

Having to exercise your willpower all the time is exhausting. It can wear out your brain and your body as well. Even your spirit. If you associate everything you see with, "No, that's not good for me," or "I can't have that," the universe hears it and makes it real.

So sometimes it is best to just accept things with gratitude, but seeking out sense pleasures that we know are not ideal is still not necessary. But don't look at it as giving in; look at it as accepting what has been put in front of you. And when you know you need to avoid something, don't label it as bad. Just acknowledge it for what it is, and move on because you know you don't need it. There are only two end-results here. We either dwell on the things we can't have to the point where the cravings and desires become unbearable and make us miserable, or we can actively and consciously choose not to indulge until the desire dissipates altogether.

If we don't focus our attention on it, if we just acknowledge it for what it is and move on, then we can bask in a newfound freedom. This is why I never suggest any drastic lifetime dietary adjustments or lifestyle adjustments. Gentle is usually more effective. When we go at something new with enthusiasm, there will be a point where eventually the enthusiasm peaks, plateaus, and then drops.

But if we take baby steps, we don't tire as quickly, and we can keep working our way up indefinitely. This is how I have been able to relate this to chronic pain. All the drastic things I did for my entire life would work for a little bit and then I would crash horribly.

But as I slowly tweak and refine my lifestyle habits, and go with the flow because I know things are always going to change, I can find peace and serenity. If a pain flare-up happens—I acknowledge it, I offer gratitude for the learning experience, I patiently wait for the flare-up to run its course—making any adjustments I might need to lessen the pain as much as possible—and then I simply move on with my life.

Just be patient and allow yourself to genuinely believe you can heal. Say it to yourself out loud all the time, and really believe it. Really put your energy into it. Put your *whole self* into it.

You may not realize it right away, but one day, the realization will hit you like a sack of bricks. You will find yourself exclaiming in awe:

"Wow! Look how far I have come!"

AFTERWORD

Now What?

Obviously, not everything in this book applies to everyone.

There is a lot of information packed in here, and it has been laid out in a framework to give you an idea of what is possible.

Determining what is right for you is a very personal process. It takes a lot of self-awareness, inner assessment, and most importantly, mindfulness.

So if you take anything away from this book, let it be this: *be mindful.*

Well, that and ... *drink hot water!*

Take notice of everything you do, how you do it, and why. When you are talking to someone, be mindful of their reactions. Put yourself in their shoes. Imagine exactly how they are feeling at that moment.

Do you find that people tend not to be very empathetic or understanding of your situation? Then

AFTERWORD

perhaps make an effort to be more empathetic and understanding of others—I promise, the karma will come full-circle eventually.

Try to be fully aware of the sensations in your body as you move about this world. Maybe your body has been trying to tell you something that you have been missing. Perhaps this could save you a lot of heartache or physical pain in the future.

Observe how you feel after trying any of the techniques suggested in this book. Your body will tell you if it is right for you or not . . . if you can listen. There is no special way to explain how to be mindful. It is something that comes to all of us naturally if we allow ourselves to tap into it.

GUT-HEALING DIET SAMPLE RECOMMENDATION

Morning Alkalizer: 6 a.m. - 11 a.m.

- 16 oz of water with a half-teaspoon of high-quality salt, lime, and stevia
- Hot lemon water
- Probiotic juice

Summertime Smoothie

- Lettuce
- Cucumber
- Zucchini
- Oil
- Herbs like cilantro, mint, basil, ginger
- Protein powder

Winter Time Soup

- Roots like burdock or daikon
- Oil
- Miso
- Bone broth

Brunch/Lunch: 11 a.m. - 2 p.m.
Vegan

- Cooked grains in a crock-pot with veggies and herbs with sea salt
- Coconut kefir

Non-Vegan

- Eggs in ghee or coconut oil. Add cultured or sauteed veggies—undercooked.
- Animal protein, raw or rare

Snack Between 3 and 4 (Try Not To, Though)

- Animal protein at beginning.

- Almond, pumpkin, or sunflower seeds; soaked and then toasted.
- Avocado with salt and dulse.
- Turkey with mayonnaise and veggies (and dip in dressing).
- Guacamole and chips (or leaf).
- Lecithin or vegetarian protein (blended with non-dairy beverage).
- Drink water with lemon and stevia for cravings (add apple cider vinegar to alkalize more).
- Mineral water with probiotics.
- Sour apple rolled in ginger with probiotics.

Dinner Before 6 p.m.

Vegetarian - Small Portion

- Slow-cooked quinoa with veggies
- Probiotic liquid
- Consider taking digestive enzymes
- Soup
- Red-skin potatoes

OR Protein Shake One Hour Before Bed

Thank you so much for purchasing this book! Now I would really appreciate your feedback. Your input will help to make the next version even better. Please leave a helpful REVIEW on Amazon, GoodReads, and/or BookBub.

I will personally read each one.

~Qat Wanders

ABOUT THE AUTHOR

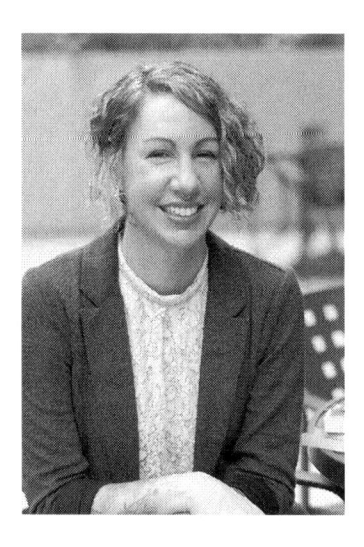

Qat Wanders is an author, editor, speaker, and writing coach. She has edited more than 4,000 books and ghostwritten over 100, including *New York Times* and *Wall Street Journal* bestsellers.

After spending almost 30 years in debilitating chronic pain, she was eventually able to heal using the four Mindful Movement Techniques™ she developed and perfected. She is a licensed Yoga Therapist and Professional Health and Wellness writer and editor. After receiving her first Yoga Alliance certification in early 2009, she has since been dedicated to customizing individual Yoga practices to suit specific needs.

While the written word is her biggest passion, Yoga is still dear to her heart because it allowed her to overcome a lifetime of chronic pain. Now she strives to share this message with the world!

With a master's degree in English Literature with an emphasis in Creative Writing and a CPE (Certified Professional Editor) certificate, Qat went on to start the Wandering Wordsmith Academy where she trains authors and editors in an online platform. This program not only trains authors to self-edit their books effectively but also helps editors create and expand a freelance editing career.

When she's not busy speaking, writing, yoga-ing, or wandering, Qat loves spending time with her daughter, Ora—a published author at ten years of age—and helping others realize their dreams of sharing their messages with the world. She now spends the majority of her time either in a cozy Colorado mountain town in the USA or a beautiful beach village in Southern India.

To find out more about Qat, her writings, her programs, and her services, please visit

www.WanderingWordsMedia.com
or find her on:

- facebook.com/qatwrites
- twitter.com/qat_wanders
- instagram.com/qatwanders
- bookbub.com/authors/qat-wanders
- goodreads.com/qat_wanders
- amazon.com/author/qatwanders

ALSO BY QAT WANDERS

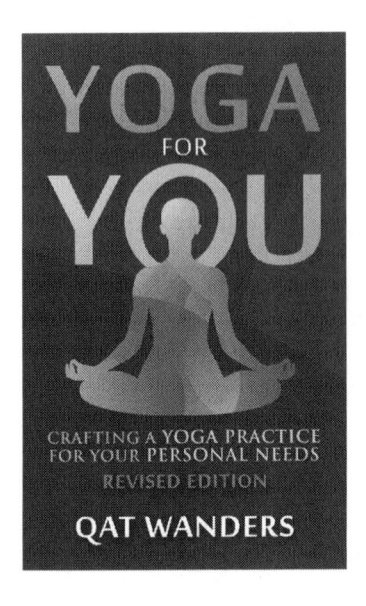

What is Yoga really all about?

Here's a hint…

…NOT stretchy pants and handstands.

Everyone has a different body and different needs. But there is a path for YOU. Physically. Mentally. Spiritually.

The methods in this book will help you find that path by giving you the tools you need to:

• Introduce 4 techniques into your physical Yoga practice to get greater results, easy and fast.

• Decide which style of Yoga will suit your needs best.

• Help you shift your mindset so you can handle the situations life throws at you with an even mind.

• Learn how to level up from the physical aspects of Yoga to approach life with more serenity and optimism.

Are you ready to go deeper?

Follow the advice here and see immediate, tangible results.

From the inside out.

Grab it on amazon!

ACKNOWLEDGMENTS

I would like to extend my deepest gratitude to everyone who assisted and supported me in the production of this book. I would like to express special thanks to: My spiritual twin, Raminyah Ingram, for keeping me in check. My mentor, Kimberly Maska, for holding me accountable. Sean Sumner and Chandler Bolt for inspiring and teaching me to do this. My fantastic cover designer, Rob Williams, and everyone on my book launch team. I could not have done this without you!

RESOURCES

BOOKS

- Boccio, Frank Jude. *Mindfulness Yoga.* Boston, Massachusetts: Wisdom Publications, 2004.
- Frawley, David. *Yoga and Ayurveda.* Twin Lakes, Wisconsin: Lotus Press, 1999.
- Gates, Donna. *The Body Ecology Diet.* Carlsbad, California: Hay House Inc., 2011.
- Hirschi, Gertrud. *Mudras: Yoga in Your Hands.* Newburyport, Massachusetts: Weiser Books, 2000.
- His Holiness, The Dalai Lama. *Freedom in Exile: The Autobiography of the Dalai Lama.* New York: Harper Collins, 1990.
- Iyengar, B.K.S. *The Tree of Yoga.* Boston,

Massachusetts: Shambhala Publications, 1988.
- Kaminoff, Leslie. *Yoga Anatomy.* Champaign, Illinois: Human Kinetics, 2007.
- Paramhansa Yogananda. *Autobiography of a Yogi.* New York: The Philosophical Library, 1946.
- Wanders, Qat. *Yoga for YOU.* Chennai, India: Happy Self-Publishing, 2017

ONLINE RESOURCES

- Bodyecology.com
- *Quiz to determine your Dosha:* http://ayurvedadosha.org/doshas/ayurveda-dosha-test#/axzz4cZ83vsOQ
- *List of chakras:* http://eocinstitute.org/meditation/secret-to-open-balanced-healed-chakras/

WANDERING WORDS
M E D I A

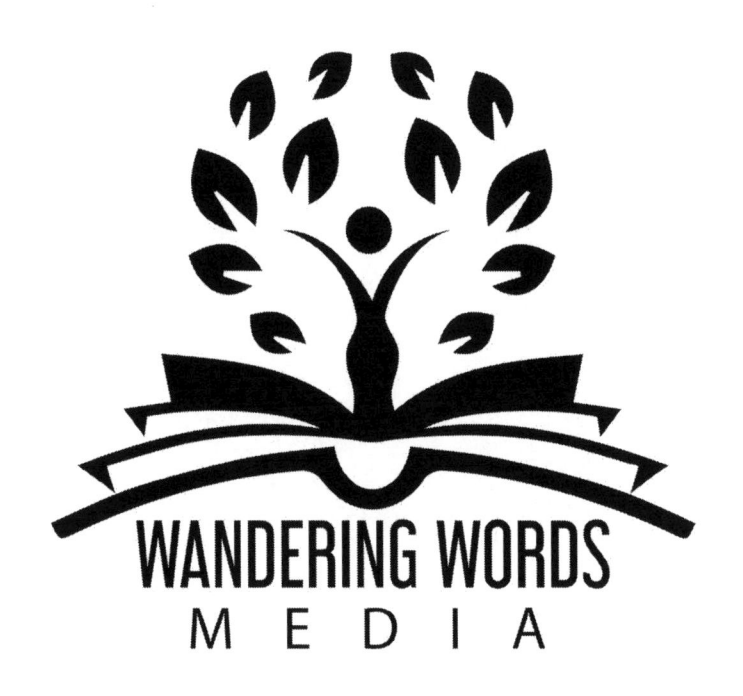

Made in the USA
Middletown, DE
10 August 2019